For two weeks now you've had daily episodes of diarrhea, abdominal pain so severe you can't think straight, and stomach bloating. You are afraid to eat and can hardly venture out of sight of a bathroom (twice in the past three days, you've barely made it). You know something is seriously wrong, but your doctor—who just returned your second call of the week—says the test results confirm her impression; there is nothing wrong with you. How can this be? You know what you feel. You're terrified it might be serious (cancer?), and you can't talk to your friends about your bowels.

If this sounds familiar, this book is for you.

Introduction

We are a team of health professionals (a clinical nutritionist, a health psychologist, and a gastroenterologist) who treat people with irritable bowel syndrome. We practice in the gastroenterology service at the Queen Elizabeth II Health Sciences Centre, a large urban teaching hospital in Nova Scotia, Canada. The three of us work together as a team because irritable bowel syndrome (also known as I.B.S.) demands a multidisciplinary approach. There are medical issues that require a gastroenterologist, nutrition issues that require a registered dietitian, and stress and coping issues that require a psychologist.

We have blended our expertise to develop a treatment plan for irritable bowel syndrome that is based on current scientific knowledge. In 10 years we have helped hundreds of patients manage their I.B.S. And now, with this book, we share our expertise with you so that you can use this treatment plan on your own.

Like most things in life, there is an upside to this and a downside.

The good news: This is a how-to manual that will help you manage your irritable bowel. Scientific studies demonstrate the effectiveness of the strategies you will learn here. If you follow our advice closely, there are good reasons to expect that your symptoms will improve.

The bad news: This is a how-to manual that will help you manage your irritable bowel. The very thing that makes this book helpful is also the thing that makes it a challenge—we require you to do the work.

This is not the kind of book that you can just read and put aside. In fact, it's more like a workbook. So if you want results, you will need to change your behavior. We will guide you as to what to change, how to change it, and how to evaluate if the change works. But, like all self-help books, you must help yourself.

As you make your way through *I.B.S. Relief,* you will see that the supporting information, self-assessments, record-keeping forms, and recommendations are all directed at discovering and treating your unique pattern of symptoms. This book would do little good if we simply presented generalities. Successful management of irritable bowel symptoms requires matching management strategies to the links between diet, stress, and symptoms that are specific to you.

So, before proceeding further, read the following statements and check the one that applies to you at this moment in time. Be honest with yourself! Don't check the statement you think you should check, or what others would want you to check. If you start by honestly assessing your readiness to change, you can avoid setting yourself up for failure and gain the maximum value from this book.

___ 1. Right now, I am ready to make changes to my diet and to practice stress management techniques.

___ 2. I am thinking about making changes to my diet and about using stress management techniques and may follow through in the next month.

___ 3. I am thinking about making changes to my diet and about using stress management techniques and may follow through in the next six months.

___ 4. I am not thinking about making changes to my diet or about using stress management techniques and won't for the next six months.

If you checked statement 1, you are ready to take action to manage your irritable bowel; *I.B.S. Relief* is ideal for you. Not only will you get the information you need, but you will also learn techniques for determining the pattern of your symptoms, identify what triggers those symptoms, and, based on this assessment, take action to control your symptoms.

We cover a lot of material in this book, so go slowly! You might find it useful to read a chapter through once to get an idea of the topics covered and the range of things that you will be asked to do. Then read the chapter again, going slowly and practicing all the strategies presented. The treatment techniques are offered "cafeteria" style, so feel free to pick and choose specific techniques that feel right and work for you. This allows you to match the techniques to your symptoms, personality, and lifestyle.

If you checked statement 2, you are preparing for change. You should find this book helpful in providing information and giving you some ideas about how to change your diet and stress management techniques. Try our suggestions but don't be surprised if you're not fully prepared to put all the effort and commitment into following through with them. Use them to help you determine the costs and benefits of trying to change your symptoms. If, having gone through the book, you decide you are ready to commit yourself, it may be helpful to go through the book again, in order to gain maximum value from the techniques.

If you checked statement 3, you are thinking about change but are not ready to commit yourself. *I.B.S. Relief* will be useful as a source of information, but don't expect big results. To make a significant impact on your symptoms, you've got to be willing to practice and use the techniques; this requires an up-front commitment. If you're not ready for this commitment, you're just not ready. Don't beat yourself up. It may help to list the advantages and disadvantages of using this book, then list the negatives of having an irritable bowel. Only when people experience significant distress about their irritable bowel—and see more advantages than disadvantages in trying to control their symptoms— are they able to commit effort into a book like this.

If you checked statement 4, we are a bit surprised that you are reading this book. Perhaps you were given *I.B.S. Relief,* and you are reading it for that person, not for yourself. If so, don't expect much relief from your symptoms. Even so, by reading this book, you will gain information that may help you decide to change sometime in the future.

We wrote *I.B.S. Relief* to accomplish two goals. First, we want to help you determine if your symptoms actually fit those of irritable bowel syndrome. Chapters 1 and 2, in particular, cover the diagnosis of an irritable bowel. If your symptoms do not point to an irritable bowel, you should see your doctor for the possibility of a bowel disease such as Crohn's disease or ulcerative colitis. Second, this book will teach you a better way of living with your particular irritable bowel symptoms. We will outline detailed changes that you can make to your diet and stress management techniques.

We provide a number of self-assessments and record-keeping forms to help you pinpoint the nature of your specific symptoms and symptom triggers. These exercises will lead you to strategies for controlling your symptoms. This can be a lengthy process, so feel free to take your time and divide the tasks into steps. It is better to work slowly and master a few points than to go quickly and learn little.

As you read *I.B.S. Relief,* be advised: Don't expect a cure. We will help you manage your symptoms and limit the frequency, intensity, and duration of irritable bowel episodes.

Still, irritable bowel syndrome tends to be chronic and is related to the way that your bowel is put together. An irritable bowel often goes through episodes of good and bad functioning. Also, stress and eating patterns fluctuate, and for some people, these factors routinely produce symptoms.

This is not meant to be bad news. Instead, it is meant to help you develop realistic expectations for this book and, for that matter, any treatment for irritable bowel syndrome. Our patients tell us they don't need a cure (though none would refuse one if it were available). They say it is sufficient to be in control of their bowel rather than feeling, as many do before they attend our clinic, that their bowel controls them.

Chapter One

What Is I.B.S.?

A t the outset, we want to clear up some terminology issues. I.B.S. is the abbreviation doctors use for irritable bowel syndrome, often when they are talking about patients. We will **not** be using I.B.S. in this book but rather the less confusing label, irritable bowel, for this disorder.

Why not I.B.S.? We have found that abbreviations can cause confusion between diseases or medical conditions. For instance, I.B.S. (irritable bowel syndrome) is often confused with I.B.D. (inflammatory bowel disease). By changing one letter, you go from having a condition (irritable bowel) that causes no serious medical complications to having a disease (inflammatory bowel) that includes serious bowel diseases like Crohn's disease and ulcerative colitis. Using the term *irritable bowel* avoids this confusion.

We also dislike using I.B.S. because the term *syndrome* is easily misunderstood. *Syndrome* tends to have a negative connotation and is often associated with mental problems or conditions. *Syndrome* actually refers to a collection of symptoms that helps diagnose certain medical (and mental) conditions. However, we don't like the word, and neither do our patients, so we will not use it again in this book.

Another confusing term that has been used to describe irritable bowel is *mucus colitis.* Thankfully, few doctors still use this term, but we feel it should be banished altogether. It frequently causes people to focus on the colitis label and think they have a serious bowel disease. As you will learn, mucus in the stool is a common symptom of an irritable bowel. As for colitis, it is a medical term that implies that the large bowel or colon is inflamed. There is no inflammation of the bowel with irritable bowel, even though some of the symptoms (diarrhea and abdominal pain) may mimic those associated with inflammation.

Diagnosing an Irritable Bowel

Irritable bowel is diagnosed by its symptoms, not a particular medical test. That's because an irritable bowel is a normal, healthy bowel, both to the naked eye and under the microscope. For some reason, though, an irritable bowel does not coordinate its functions normally. It is also extra sensitive to food, stress, and other stimulants. However, irritable bowel does **not** lead to bowel cancer or other serious bowel diseases such as colitis, Crohn's disease, or ulcers. (See appendix 1, page 145, for information on how the bowel and entire gastrointestinal tract normally works.)

Doctors look for a specific pattern of symptoms when diagnosing an irritable bowel. If you have had at least three of the six most common symptoms for more than three months—without symptoms that might indicate bowel disease (see page 16)—then a "positive" diagnosis of irritable bowel can be made. The more symptoms you experience, the more likely it is that you have an irritable bowel.

Common Symptoms of an Irritable Bowel

- Abdominal pain for at least three months. It can be present continuously, but more often it is intermittent (on and off over time).
- Increased frequency of bowel movements when the pain occurs. Alternatively, infrequent bowel movements (constipation) may be experienced at other times.
- Increased looseness of stool when the abdominal pain is felt. At other times, the stool form may be hard or constipated.
- Mucus in the stool.
- A sensation of incomplete emptying of the rectum after going to the bathroom.
- A bloated or distended feeling in the abdomen.

To rule out serious disease, doctors also usually perform a physical examination, along with a few simple blood tests. Experienced doctors need very few tests to diagnose irritable bowel, especially when at least three of the symptoms are present and there are no unusual symptoms.

Although distressing at times, irritable bowel symptoms do not mean there is anything wrong with the intestine. The frequency and severity of the symptoms as well do not indicate that anything harmful will happen or develop in the bowel.

What Symptoms Are Not Related to an Irritable Bowel?

The most important symptom to watch for is blood in the stool. Bleeding does not occur with an irritable bowel. If you see blood in your stool, you need to see your doctor. The bleeding may not signal a serious cause, but it is not a symptom of an irritable bowel.

Do your bowel symptoms cause you to wake from sleep? If so, this is very unusual with irritable bowel. Bowel symptoms arise from bowel activity, and your bowel "goes to sleep" when you do. Although waking from sleep with bowel symptoms and pain can occur at times, it usually indicates an underlying disease of the bowel.

Finally, fever and unexplained weight loss are also not related to an irritable bowel, so we urge you to see your doctor if you have these symptoms.

Does an Irritable Bowel Cause Other Problems?

People with an irritable bowel can have a number of symptoms in other parts of the body. The following symptoms cannot be used to diagnose an irritable bowel, but they are commonly associated with irritable bowel. (See page 13 for more information.)

- Urinary problems are quite common, and usually involve feeling the need to pass urine more frequently, often with urgency.
- Migraine headaches appear to be associated with an irritable bowel in some people.

- Painful sexual intercourse for women, presumably because the surrounding pelvic structures, like the bladder and bowel, are also oversensitive or "irritable."
- Fatigue is very common. Generally its source is unclear, but in context with the common symptoms of irritable bowel, fatigue can often be linked with an irritable bowel.
- Heartburn is also frequently experienced by people with an irritable bowel. This may reflect the increased bowel sensitivity, which can affect the esophagus and stomach and cause heartburn or indigestion. However, there are many other causes for heartburn and indigestion, so you should see your doctor if you suffer mostly with these symptoms.
- Fibromyalgia—a poorly understood disorder that causes chronic muscle pain, fatigue, memory problems, and other symptoms—is reportedly more common in people with an irritable bowel.

Who Gets an Irritable Bowel?

Studies over the last 10 years have led to a much better understanding of irritable bowel. We now know that irritable bowel usually strikes young, healthy adults. Many people start to experience symptoms before they turn 30. In fact, if you are over 40 and are suddenly having irritable bowel symptoms for the first time, you should see your doctor. A recent intestinal infection could be the culprit. Research shows that an infection can cause inflammation of the bowel, which can result in a prolonged disturbance of the bowel—even after the inflammation heals and the offending organism is cleared from the body. Bowel function gradually returns to normal in most but not all cases.

As mentioned earlier, irritable bowel symptoms arise from disordered coordination of the bowel and because the bowel is more sensitive than normal. An estimated 10 to 15 percent of the population in North America have an irritable bowel. Actually, with so much activity taking place in the gut during and between meals, it is surprising that irritable bowel isn't more prevalent. Most people appear to be completely oblivious to intestinal activity. Even so, irritable bowel is the second leading cause of absenteeism from work and school after the common cold, according to researchers at Tufts University in Boston.

All told, irritable bowel affects twice as many women as men, particularly in Western cultures such as North America and Western Europe. Limited studies around the globe have found people in parts of Africa, China, and India with irritable bowel. Interestingly, in India more men report symptoms than women, though we do not know why this occurs there but nowhere else.

Irritable bowel symptoms do not occur persistently in an individual. They appear to come and go over time—often triggered or worsened by dietary factors and stress. About half of the population with irritable bowel seeks medical attention. Not surprisingly, a visit to the doctor usually depends on the frequency and severity of symptoms.

Women and men generally experience the same symptoms, though abdominal bloating is more common in women. Both men and women see doctors if they have a lot of abdominal pain or multiple bowel symptoms. On the other hand, men are more likely to seek medical attention if they are having a lot of diarrhea with urgency.

For anyone, the fear of losing control of the bowel can be very disabling and stressful. Sometimes the diarrhea and urgency to pass stool can be so intense it causes incontinence or the loss of bowel control. If you have this problem you should see your doctor. Many treatments are available to control fecal incontinence, especially if the incontinence is mainly with loose, watery stools.

If You've Been Told Your Symptoms Are "All in Your Head"

Irritable bowel symptoms are real. They occur because the bowel is not working in a normal, coordinated manner. Unfortunately, many doctors have led patients to believe that because no abnormalities can be found in either X rays or blood tests, their symptoms must be "in their head." This is incorrect! And we hope this book dispels this myth.

Understanding that the intestines are more sensitive may actually serve as a useful guide for you to help monitor other aspects of your life. What will follow in subsequent chapters is a discussion as to how you can use the symptoms of an irritable bowel to adjust your diet and to evaluate the effects of stress on your body. An irritable bowel may actually serve as an "early warning system," so that when you ingest a diet that may not be ideal for your body (for example, high fat or high caffeine intake), your gut will let you know it doesn't like these foods. Perhaps even more importantly, this heightened sensitivity of the gut may help you to identify when you are experiencing certain situations or life events as being stressful because of the increase in your intestinal symptoms. Adjusting what you are doing when you experience irritable bowel symptoms may help to minimize or alleviate the stressful conditions in a more positive and healthy manner. You will learn more about these techniques when you read about diet in chapters 4, 5, and 6 and the effects of stress on an irritable bowel in chapters 7 and 8.

It's not uncommon for patients to look to medications or over-the-counter preparations such as laxatives to relieve their symptoms. Unfortunately, long-term use can actually damage the gut and aggravate problems. That's why it is best to avoid relying on drugs to manage your symptoms and instead learn the techniques in this book.

No single drug will treat all the symptoms of irritable bowel. And any attempt to develop such a drug will probably never be successful. The majority of people with irritable bowel experience symptoms off and on throughout their lives. It would not make sense for these healthy individuals to take drugs for 30 or 40 years, especially when potential side effects and long-term effects are difficult to study.

Take a few moments now to complete the questionnaire on the next few pages. This questionnaire will help you identify your irritable bowel symptoms and help you begin to link symptoms to treatment. Chapter 2 will elaborate on some of the concepts we have discussed and help you to confirm if you do indeed have an irritable bowel.

Do I Have an Irritable Bowel?

For each question, please check the answer that applies. At the end of the questionnaire, score your answers to see if you have an irritable bowel.

1. In the past three months have you had continuous or repeated discomfort or pain in your lower abdomen? (If No, skip to question 5.) ....Yes   No

2. Is this discomfort or pain relieved by a bowel movement? ......Yes   No

3. Is this discomfort or pain associated with a change in the frequency of bowel movement (for instance, having more or fewer bowel movements)? ....Yes   No

4. Is this discomfort or pain associated with a change in the consistency of the stool (for instance, softer or harder)? ....Yes   No

5. Would you say that at least one-fourth of the occasions or days in the last three months you have had any of the following? (Check all that apply.)

____ Fewer than three bowel movements a week (0–2).
____ More than three bowel movements a day (4 or more).
____ Hard or lumpy stools.
____ Loose or watery stools.
____ Straining during a bowel movement.
____ Urgency—having to rush to the bathroom for a bowel movement.
____ Feeling of incomplete emptying after a bowel movement.
____ Passing mucus (whitish material) during a bowel movement.
____ Abdominal fullness, bloating, or swelling.

6. If you have had loose or watery stools, would you say that it occurred with more than three-fourths of your total bowel movements in the past three months? ....Yes   No

7. If you have had over three bowel movements a day in the past three months, would you say that it occurred more than half of the days? ....Yes   No

8. In the past three months, have you noticed a large amount of stools per evacuation? ....Yes   No

9. Over the past six months, have you had continuous or frequently recurring pain in your abdomen? (If you are female, this should not be related to your menstrual cycle or period.) (If No, skip to question 11.) ....Yes   No

10. Has this pain interfered with your daily activities from time to time? (For example, inability to work or a decrease in social events.) ....Yes   No

11. Do you suffer from frequent headaches, or have you been told by your doctor that you have migraine headaches? ....Yes   No

Adapted with permission from: D.A. Drossman, et al., "Research Diagnostic Questions for Functional Gastrointestinal Disorders," in *The Functional Gastrointestinal Disorders* (McLean VA: Delnon & Associates, 1994), 341–42.

12. Do you suffer from fatigue or feeling very tired most days such that it interferes with your daily activities such as being able to work or take part in social activities? . . . . .Yes   No

13. Do you suffer from recurrent muscle and joint aches or pains, or have you been told by your doctor that you have a condition called fibromyalgia? . . . . .Yes   No

14. If you are female, in the past three months have you suffered with discomfort or pain during sexual intercourse? . . . . . . .Yes   No

15. In the past three months have you had to rush to pass urine or feel that you have to frequently pass urine while awake during the day? . . . . .Yes   No

16. Do you ever see blood in your bowel movements? . . . . .Yes   No

17. Do you wake out of a deep sleep at night with your bowel symptoms or with abdominal discomfort or pain? . . . . .Yes   No

18. When you are troubled by your bowel symptoms, do you ever experience fever (>100°F or 38°C)? .Yes   No

19. In the past three months, have you noticed weight loss without attempting to restrict or change your diet? . . . . .Yes   No

20. Do you vomit when you have abdominal discomfort or pain? . .Yes   No

21. If you have answered Yes to any of questions 1 to 9, are you over 40 years old *and* experiencing these symptoms for the first time ever in your life? . . . . .Yes   No

Scoring the Questionnaire

You have an irritable bowel if:

- you answer *yes* to question 1 and *yes* to questions 2, 3, or 4, and
- you have two or more responses to question 5.

If you answered *yes* on question 5 to items 1, 3, 5, and/or 7, then constipation is a main problem and you will be helped by increasing dietary fiber in your diet. (See, "The High-Fiber Diet" in chapter 6.)

If you answered *yes* to questions 6, 7, and/or 8, then diarrhea is a major problem and you may not find increasing dietary fiber especially helpful; if you try a high-fiber diet, you should introduce fiber very gradually. Other possible diet adjustments are important to know because certain foods and beverages can worsen diarrhea. (See chapter 5.)

If you have answered *yes* on question 5 to item 9, then you have problems with abdominal bloating. (See, "The Low Gassy Foods Diet" in chapter 6.)

You may have a more serious bowel disorder if you answered *yes* to any of questions 16 to 21. If you answered *yes* to *any* of these questions, you should see your doctor!

If you answered *yes* to questions 9 *and* 10, then you have significant problems with abdominal pain. (See chapter 9.)

If you answered *yes* to questions 11 to 15, then you have some of the common non-bowel symptoms associated with an irritable bowel. These symptoms can all be treated by your doctor, but you may find this book helpful, since improving the bowel symptoms of an irritable bowel often helps decrease the severity of associated non-bowel symptoms.

Chapter Two

How Do I Know I Have an Irritable Bowel?

As you now know, irritable bowel is not diagnosed by doing lots of tests, since no test can make a positive diagnosis of irritable bowel. Tests can only exclude diseases that may be causing your symptoms. The symptoms themselves are used to diagnose an irritable bowel.

In this chapter we will spend more time explaining and reviewing some of the concepts already introduced, plus provide more information about how a diagnosis is actually made.

Pain: The Number One Symptom

It can be frightening and confusing to experience the symptoms of an irritable bowel—especially pain. From early on, we have learned that pain is not good; something must be wrong. Unfortunately, recurring bouts of abdominal pain for at least three months are the main symptom of an irritable bowel. Pain is also the most common reason we seek a doctor's advice. But pain does not always mean there is a serious disease. This is especially true with irritable bowel.

The pain associated with an irritable bowel is often located in the lower part of the abdomen below the belly button but can be felt throughout the abdomen. The pain occurs because of the heightened sensitivity of the bowel. After a bowel movement, though, the bowel relaxes and the pain usually goes away, often returning a few minutes later. This is quite characteristic of irritable bowel and is less commonly seen with bowel diseases. If there is a serious disease such as colitis or inflammation of the bowel, the pain often lingers though the intensity may decrease. This is because the pain is due to the inflammation of the bowel, which continues even though the contractions to cause a bowel movement have stopped.

Although pain is normal with irritable bowel, it does not mean that you cannot or should not do anything about it. Changing your diet and practicing stress management techniques (explained later in this book) will help ease your symptoms, as will following the advice in chapter 9, which details the best ways to manage pain. Still, you shouldn't hesitate to see your doctor about abdominal pain, especially if it has surfaced recently, is very severe, or you have never experienced a similar pain.

The Other Diagnostic Symptoms

When you are having abdominal pain, you may notice that there is a change in your stool pattern. Bowel movements occur more frequently, usually becoming more liquid and watery. A typical pattern is the onset of abdominal pain, followed shortly by a somewhat formed bowel movement with temporary relief of the pain. This is followed by repeated spasms of pain, with increasingly looser bowel movements (more and more liquid in the stool). These "attacks" of pain and frequent trips to the bathroom often occur over several hours, leaving many people quite drained and exhausted.

Another common symptom of an irritable bowel is an irregular pattern of defecation occurring at least 25 percent of the time. For instance, you might have a regular bowel movement every day, but every fourth week your bowel movements are either more constipated or looser and diarrhea-like. In fact, having isolated episodes of irregular bowel function—interspersed with normal bowel function—is more typical with an irritable bowel than with bowel diseases. When the bowel is inflamed, which occurs with Crohn's disease, colitis, and other bowel diseases, the change in bowel habits usually lasts several weeks until the inflammation settles. This irregular bowel function usually distinguishes irritable bowel symptoms from more serious bowel disease.

The presence of mucus in the stool is another symptom of an irritable bowel. Many people believe mucus in the stool indicates they have a serious bowel disease, such as colitis. In fact, mucus alone (without blood) is a common finding with irritable bowel patients; **not** patients with colitis. People with colitis see blood mixed with the mucus in the stool.

A normal product of the bowel, mucus is produced by the intestine as a lubricant. In individuals with an irritable bowel, however, extra mucus is produced. This mucus is particularly visible if the stool is loose, but it also occasionally occurs with a constipated bowel motion. On rare occasions, patients may even pass mucus alone without stool.

Another common symptom of an irritable bowel, especially if you are constipated, is abdominal bloating or swelling. The bloating, which can often be quite pronounced, is usually worse later in the day and after eating. It frequently disappears or improves significantly overnight during sleep but then recurs the following day in a similar pattern. This type of variable abdominal distension is seen only with an irritable bowel. Serious conditions such as a fluid collection in the abdomen or a tumor growth will cause abdominal swelling, but it does not come and go over a 24-hour period.

Finally, the sixth common symptom of an irritable bowel is a sensation of incomplete emptying of the rectum after defecation. This often causes a great deal of distress and concern. People frequently feel that their bowel motions are incomplete, and they strain excessively to try to pass stool. This symptom again reflects the irritability or, perhaps more appropriately, the increased sensitivity of the gut. In most people with this symptom, the rectum has indeed emptied completely, and the feeling of incomplete emptying is a "false" sensation caused by an oversensitive rectum.

Other Symptoms Associated With an Irritable Bowel

As mentioned in chapter 1, irritable bowel can also be associated with symptoms in other parts of the body, not just the intestines. Several studies have shown that people with an irritable bowel have more frequent symptoms of heartburn. This might reflect the generalized increased sensitivity of the gut, which includes the stomach and esophagus.

Another non-bowel symptom frequently noted by people with an irritable bowel is fatigue. Recent studies have shown that many people with severe irritable bowel symptoms have disturbed sleep patterns, and it may be this disruption that further aggravates or accentuates a tendency to having irritable bowel symptoms. Fatigue may also point to more serious psychological problems such as depression (see chapters 8 and 10). Sometimes irritable bowel symptoms will improve as measures to reduce fatigue succeed.

Bladder or urinary problems are also associated with irritable bowel. There may be times when you feel you have to pass urine more frequently or experience a sudden urge to pass urine. You may even feel like you are about to lose control. Yet when you actually urinate, there may not be much urine at all. The source of this sensation is not known; however, it may be that an irritable bowel causes a generalized sensitivity of the smooth muscle that lines the bowel and bladder. This same effect may be the reason migraine headaches are linked to irritable bowel, since smooth muscle also lines the blood vessels that cause the throbbing effect of migraine headaches. Still, the factors that lead to migraine headache are much more complicated, and at present, the reason why migraine and irritable bowel are associated has not been resolved.

It's common for women to notice that their irritable bowel symptoms occur around the time of their menstrual cycle. If this happens to you, try your best to avoid any other "triggers" that can bring on or worsen bowel symptoms such as certain foods and stress or anxiety. (More on this throughout the book.) The combination of these "triggers" will lead to even more intense symptoms during your period. Women with irritable bowel symptoms can also be troubled by painful intercourse. This symptom may reflect the increased sensitivity of the other organs in the pelvis, including the bladder and bowel.

Some people with irritable bowel also suffer from a condition called fibromyalgia. This condition could be called the "irritable bowel of the muscles." For some reason, muscles and tendons appear to have increased sensitivity and areas of localized tenderness and pain. Again, pain is the major symptom, and it can aggravate irritable bowel symptoms. With fibromyalgia, pain can be felt in the muscles of the abdominal wall under the skin. This pain can be quite intense and persistent because the abdominal muscles are large, powerful muscles that we use all day (like our back muscles). When they become sensitive and prone to pain, it can be very difficult to achieve pain relief. Abdominal muscles are called "postural muscles" because they are used to support the body and maintain posture. These muscles are used even when we are resting, such as sitting in a chair or lying down. Even shifting your weight to roll on your side may trigger the pain. Because of all these factors, the abdominal pain can be persistent and keep relapsing. Chapter 9 covers pain management techniques.

Pinpointing Your Symptoms

As you explore whether irritable bowel is indeed the reason for the symptoms you are experiencing, it will help to complete the checklist on the next page for your next doctor's visit. Irritable bowel can usually be diagnosed without lots of tests. However, common symptoms of irritable bowel can mimic or overlap those of other bowel conditions or diseases.

If you have any concerns or do not feel that your symptoms exactly fit those for an irritable bowel, then you should seek the advice of your doctor. Not only will the checklist be helpful in confirming or refuting a diagnosis of irritable bowel, it will serve as an up-to-date list of your symptoms.

Making It Fit: Identifying Your Symptoms and Patterns of Functioning

For this book to be useful, you need to be able to see improvements in your own symptoms. It is not enough for us to talk about general issues concerning irritable bowel, diet, and stress. We must help you identify the specific symptoms that you experience, and their connection to diet, stress, and other factors.

In our clinical work, this is straightforward; we simply assess patients and their circumstances. We cannot do this in a book. You must assess yourself.

Symptom List (to Show Your Doctor)

1. Pain in the lower half of the belly or abdomen. . . . . .Yes   No
2. Pain present for weeks. . . . . .Yes   No
3. Abdominal pain is relieved by having a bowel motion. . . . . .Yes   No
4. Bowels are looser when I have the pain. .Yes   No
5. I have more frequent bowel motions with the pain. . . . . .Yes   No
6. I am constipated when I have the pain. . . . . .Yes   No
7. I have to strain to make my bowels work. . . . . .Yes   No
8. I have to rush to the bathroom for fear of losing control
   of my bowels. . . . . .Yes   No
9. I feel I don't finish when I do have a bowel motion. . . . . .Yes   No
10. I see mucus (slime) when I have a bowel motion. . . . . .Yes   No
11. I feel bloated and have swelling of my belly. . . . . .Yes   No
12. I feel tired all the time. . . . . .Yes   No
13. I have frequent headaches. . . . . .Yes   No
14. I frequently have muscle and joint aching. . . . . .Yes   No
15. I have to rush when I pass urine. . . . . .Yes   No
16. I have trouble sleeping. . . . . .Yes   No

Bowel Symptoms I Must Tell My Doctor About!

1. I see blood in my stool or bowel motions. . . . . .Yes   No
2. I see black bowel motions. . . . . .Yes   No
3. I have noted a fever. . . . . .Yes   No
My temperature was: _____.
4. I have been noticing weight loss without being on
   a weight-reducing diet. . . . . .Yes   No
   I have lost _____ lbs. in the past _____ months.
5. I have noticed the pain can wake me out of a deep sleep
   at night. . . . . .Yes   No
6. I vomit with the pain. . . . . .Yes   No
7. I have seen blood or black colored material when I have
   vomited. . . . . .Yes   No

One of the best ways to monitor and identify your symptoms is to complete the diary starting on page 19 over a 1-week period. The information you collect during the week will help you become familiar with the specifics of your symptoms and begin to evaluate connections between diet, stress, and your symptoms. These insights will be particularly helpful as you read the chapters on diet and stress.

Recording sometimes unpleasant symptoms for a week may

seem like a long time when you want relief, but we find that in order to best identify connections between stress, diet, and symptoms, a week is the minimum time. This is because the connection between diet, stress, and symptoms is not necessarily immediate and clear. As you will learn, stress that occurs one day may not affect the bowel for several days. Furthermore, it may not affect the bowel to the same degree, and in the same way, each time. General feelings and worries can also influence how you experience your bowel symptoms. If you are worried that your symptoms are due to cancer, your symptoms will cause more alarm than if you realize they are due to a pizza you ate.

A symptom diary is necessary because you need to be able to collect enough information to be able to stand back and observe patterns. Often we see people who can't see the forest for the trees; they tell us, "I was really stressed Tuesday at work but my bowel was fine. On Thursday I couldn't stand the pain, but everything was calm—I had no stress." Similar delayed patterns occur for diet as well.

We want to emphasize the importance of you doing this assessment. Successfully managing irritable bowel symptoms requires matching management strategies to symptoms and understanding the links between diet, stress, and symptoms that are specific to you. All individuals are unique. Plus, while we have expertise in the medical, nutritional, and psychological aspects of irritable bowel, you are the expert on you!

In the chapters that follow, we will ask you to refer to your symptom diary in order to help you assess yourself and plan treatment. This will make it much easier for you to choose which strategies will best fit your situation. We will ask you to fill out a diary again after you have completed the book. This will allow you to evaluate how successful the program has been and allow you to compare yourself from before to after.

How to Complete a Symptom Diary

To complete the diary, first choose a time each day to fill it out. Most people prefer the end of the day, which tends to be calmer, so you can think clearly and the day's events are still fresh on the mind. Write down the day and time that you fill in the diary.

Then, record any irritable bowel symptoms you experience and their severity. Try to summarize each symptom you had that day in one or two words (see the list on page 16) and, beside each symptom, write the number that corresponds to the severity of the symptom. Use a rating between 1 and 10, where 1 means not at all severe, 5 means moderately severe, and 10 means extremely severe.

Next, consider your diet. Try to identify any foods, or patterns of eating, that you suspect may trigger your symptoms. Did you eat anything that may have upset you? Did you skip any meals or eat too fast?

It's not the easiest to identify possible diet-related triggers, so don't worry if you have trouble at this point. The chapters on diet and stress will help you learn how to be more precise in your assessment of symptom triggers. Right now, we simply want you to start thinking about possible triggers. Jot down anything that you suspect is a food trigger. Otherwise, make a brief note about what you ate.

Next, rate your daily stress level using a scale between 1 and 10 (1 for not at all stressed, 5 for moderately stressed, and 10 for extremely stressed). If you were stressed at all, make a brief note about the source of stress.

Sometimes people become so accustomed to stress that they have trouble identifying it. Don't worry if this is the case; just ask yourself, what was stressful about today? Again, at this stage we just want to help you begin to identify patterns.

Finally, we want you to identify any feelings and worries associated with your symptoms that day. In the last column write down the feelings caused by your symptoms, such as anxiety, frustration, and sadness. Also, if you are aware of any worrisome thoughts associated with your symptoms, write them here. This will be helpful for you to determine how your thoughts and concerns can impact on the severity or onset of your symptoms.

Do your best to complete the symptom diary each day. It may seem awkward at first, but after two or three days you will get the hang of it. Almost everyone who completes a diary for a whole week learns something important about their irritable bowel.

ENLARGE THIS RECORD TO 200% ON YOUR COPIER

Symptom Diary

	Monday	Tuesday	Wednesday
Date and Time			
Symptoms and Severity (1=not at all severe; 10=extremely severe)			
Food Triggers			
Stress Level (1=no stress; 10=extreme stress)			
Feelings and Worries			

19

ENLARGE THIS RECORD TO 200% ON YOUR COPIER

Symptom Diary

Date and Time

Symptoms and Severity
(1=not at all severe; 10=extremely severe)

Food Triggers

Stress Level
(1=no stress; 10=extreme stress)

Feelings and Worries

Thursday

Friday

Saturday

Sunday

Chapter Three

What Causes Irritable Bowel?

A great deal of research in the last decade has been directed at discovering what causes an irritable bowel. We have learned a lot, but unfortunately, important questions are still unanswered.

For many years it was thought that an irritable bowel was caused by abnormal "motility," which describes the coordinated contractions of the bowel that move digested food and gas through the intestines as part of the digestion process. The bowel is like a big muscle, and fecal material is moved through the bowel by a special type of muscular movement called peristaltic movements. These contractions can be compared with the action that is necessary to pull a cord through the waistband of a pair of sweatpants or a hood. People with an irritable bowel have abnormal coordination of these bowel contractions at times. However, research into these motility abnormalities did not show a good correlation between the abnormal contractions and bowel symptoms. Another problem is the erratic muscle contraction patterns of the bowel, particularly in the large intestine. These erratic patterns were also found in people without irritable bowel, so abnormal motility did not explain all the irritable bowel symptoms. This led investigators to look to other theories.

Recent studies suggest that another problem may be an abnormally heightened sensitivity of the gut, particularly the intestines. (Some sufferers also have a more sensitive stomach and esophagus as well.) In research studies, people with irritable bowel experienced much more pain than others when their bowel was distended with a balloon.

It was further shown that people with irritable bowel have such heightened sensitivity that they feel certain muscle contraction patterns in the intestine as painful or unpleasant. These same contraction patterns go unnoticed by people without irritable bowel. This discovery has revolutionized our thinking as to the underlying causes of irritable bowel.

It appears that individuals with irritable bowel actually perceive and react to normal day-to-day activity in the gut such as food digestion, defecation, and movement of food waste through the intestine. This suggests that irritable bowel is probably at the high end of a spectrum of intestinal awareness. Normal stimulation of an irritable bowel can produce abnormal overreactions— the cardinal symptoms of irritable bowel (pain, altered bowel habits, mucus, bloating, and sensations of incomplete rectal emptying). Stressful events can also generate symptoms.

The Infection Connection

Beyond an overly sensitive gut, we know that irritable bowel can result from an infection of the intestines. Irritable bowel strikes approximately 30 percent of people who experience a severe diarrheal illness caused by an infection. Irritable bowel symptoms can persist for years after the infection has cleared, or they may gradually fade over several months when a more normal bowel habit returns.

Research into postinfection irritable bowel has found that the nerves in the gut are sensitized by an infection and develop a "memory" of the disordered bowel function that is present when infected. So even after the infection is gone, symptoms similar to those caused by an infection persist (diarrhea, pain and cramping, mucus, and a feeling of incomplete rectal emptying). Again, symptoms caused by an infection can, in the short term, mimic those of an irritable bowel. This is why your doctor cannot make a diagnosis of an irritable bowel until the symptoms have been present for more than three months.

The Brain's Role

Research studies of nerve function have found that there may also be differences within the brain in people with irritable bowel and the way they "experience" bowel symptoms. We know from several studies that the degree of distress people are experiencing will influence whether they seek medical advice for their irritable bowel symptoms. It may be that these individuals magnify the intensity of the bowel symptoms experienced by the brain, due to the distress they are having. Only about half of all people with irritable bowel go to doctors with their complaints. The people who appear to be under less stress are not worried or as concerned about their symptoms and do not seek medical attention.

Studies have also shown that loss of sleep will increase the intensity of irritable bowel symptoms, suggesting the brain can modulate these symptoms markedly. To further support this link between the brain and the gut, other studies have shown people with irritable bowel experience definite abnormal contractions in the gut when they are placed in stressful situations. More research is necessary, but it is clear that the heightened sensitivity of the gut stems from underlying problems in the gut's nervous system or altered nerve connections between the brain and gut, which lead to these abnormal responses to food and stress as well as other triggers.

Using Science to Your Benefit

Though researchers do not yet know the exact forces that cause irritable bowel, their work has led to better and better strategies for managing symptoms. For instance, understanding that the intestines are more sensitive than normal may be useful as you monitor important aspects of your life.

Think of your irritable bowel as an "early warning system." Your gut will let you know when your diet is less than ideal (for example, consuming large amounts of high-fat foods or caffeine). Perhaps even more importantly, this heightened sensitivity of the gut may help you identify when you are experiencing stressful situations or life events so that you can quickly respond in a positive and healthy manner.

Chapter Four

Want Relief? Start With a Healthy Diet

Adopting a healthy diet is the first step to managing an irritable bowel. This does not mean you will be expected to become "virtuous" with your food choices (which is what many people think dietitians demand when they recommend a healthy diet). Instead, the advice in this and the next two chapters is based on science and a mix of professional and personal experience.

You see, dietitians tend to be drawn to their profession for the very reason that they like food. And while most dietitians follow a healthy diet, they also enjoy the occasional pizza and piece of cheesecake. We make this point in the beginning so that you understand that our nutrition recommendations reflect optimal strategies for managing irritable bowel symptoms tempered with the appreciation that food is an important if not focal part of life.

First, though, a word of caution: no magic food or diet will cure your irritable bowel. You will hear claims that if you follow a special diet (often restrictive) or consume a specific product (often expensive), your irritable bowel will be cured. However, irritable bowel is never really cured. The symptoms are treated or managed through a variety of nutritional, psychological, and medical strategies as presented in this book.

When you have an irritable bowel, there is a strong relationship between what you eat and how you feel. Instead of "you are what you eat," it should be "you feel what you eat." You probably know this already because you have had symptoms after eating certain foods. And you may have eliminated these foods from your diet only to have your symptoms persist. Unfortunately, there is more to managing symptoms of an irritable bowel than removing foods from the diet. Read on, and we will take the mystery out of the malady.

In these three chapters on nutrition, we will educate you on how to manage your irritable bowel symptoms through diet. There are three distinct steps to pursue. First, you will need to adopt a healthy diet. Then, as you will learn in the next chapter, you will need to adjust your eating habits (in many ways, your lifestyle) based on the diet-related causes of irritable bowel symptoms. These two steps are important because you need adequate nutrition to feel well, function normally, and cope with stress. Also, you need to know the eating habits that may be triggering your symptoms in order to manage your condition effectively. Finally, in chapter 6, you will learn how to control you irritable bowel symptoms with a specific diet(s). Following this three-step process is critical to managing your symptoms. If you skip the first step or second one you will be disappointed, because any efforts you make will be less effective.

One final word before proceeding: There is a lot of material in this chapter and the next two. You may want to read each chapter through once from beginning to end, then go back and work through each section again, this time more slowly.

Healthy Eating: You Feel What You Eat

To start off, we want to make the point that a healthy diet is a way of life or a lifestyle, not something you do one day (or week) and then not the next. This is important to understand. As you will see, managing your irritable bowel symptoms will require you to make and stick with changes if you want to feel better. These changes may be challenging, but we are confident that you will find the rewards worth the effort. You will be in control of your symptoms.

Our discussion on healthy eating centers on the Food Guide Pyramid, which is designed to help healthy people, ages two years and older, choose a healthy diet.

The Food Guide Pyramid

The Food Guide Pyramid* provides direction on how to choose a healthy diet. It emphasizes choosing foods from five major food groups shown in the three lower sections of the Pyramid (see page 28).

All types of foods are represented on the Pyramid, even those that should be eaten sparingly, such as fats and sugars. Each food group provides specific nutrients, but not all of the nutrients you need. For your health you need to choose a variety of foods from all of the food groups.

The Pyramid guides you on how many servings to choose from each food group. If your energy needs are small (for example, you have a sedentary lifestyle), you should stick to the lower number of servings in each food group to moderate your energy (calorie) intake. If your energy needs are on the high side (for example, you are very active and/or in your teens or 20s), you can choose the maximum serving amounts. Most people require the mid-range of servings from each food group. Everyone should eat, on average, at least the minimum number of servings from each food group, daily.

When we talk about healthy diet we aren't referring to a single meal or one day. We are talking about your diet over several days. Some days you simply may eat more vegetables than others, or more or less fat than others. If you are eating healthy foods, the varied intake should balance out over several days.

Pyramid Concepts

Variety Selecting a variety of foods within and among the different food groups will ensure that you eat a variety of nutrients. This is very important to a healthy diet.

Variety is achieved by selecting a variety of foods at each meal. Meals with variety contain three or more food groups (see the Food Guide Pyramid). For example, a breakfast of cereal, low-fat milk, and juice represents three food groups. Lunch consisting of a sandwich filled with a lean meat, a glass of milk or yogurt, and a piece of fruit covers four food groups. A supper of lean meat,

---

*See appendix 2 for Canada's Food Guide to Healthy Eating and a brief discussion comparing the Canadian and American food guides.

The Food Guide Pyramid

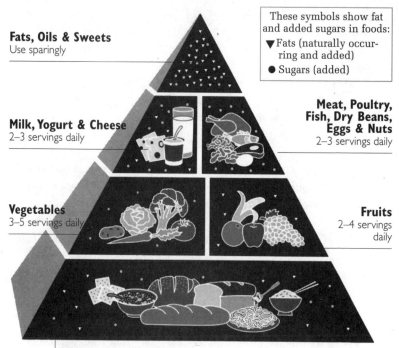

These symbols show fat and added sugars in foods:
▼ Fats (naturally occurring and added)
● Sugars (added)

Fats, Oils & Sweets
Use sparingly

Milk, Yogurt & Cheese
2–3 servings daily

Meat, Poultry, Fish, Dry Beans, Eggs & Nuts
2–3 servings daily

Vegetables
3–5 servings daily

Fruits
2–4 servings daily

Breads, Cereals, Rice & Pasta
6–11 servings daily

vegetables, whole-wheat bread or pasta or rice, a glass of milk, and a piece of fruit covers five food groups.

Balance Eat appropriate amounts of food for you. The Pyramid recommends a range of servings for each group. The number of servings you require is based on age, gender, size, and level of physical activity.

Balancing is a useful concept for allowing flexibility in your diet. You may choose to balance your eating by having a small lunch when you know that supper will be higher in calories. Or you can choose pasta in a tomato sauce instead of cream sauce if you would like to have an appetizer or a dessert. Some nutrition professionals refer to this type of balancing as "trading off." Trading off will help you to follow the Food Guide Pyramid while enjoying flexibility in selecting many types of foods.

Moderation We know that you've heard this term before. Some substances should be in our diet in moderate amounts: fats, cholesterol, salt, sugars, caffeine, and alcohol. Choose a variety of foods to meet your nutrient needs while making sure that you do not consume too much of the above substances. For example, to moderate your fat intake, choose low-fat foods most often such as a baked or mashed potato rather than fried, or a bagel instead of a croissant.

Pyramid Particulars

Breads, Cereals, Rice, & Pasta Group The bottom level of the Pyramid contains foods from different grains—the breads, cereals, rice, and pasta group. Your body requires the most of your food choices from these foods each day. This food group has plenty of complex carbohydrates (your body likes these starchy foods for fuel, particularly if they are low in fat), fiber, and B vitamins.

This food group is particularly important to people with an irritable bowel for two reasons. First, cereals and grains are a good source of fiber. Choosing whole-grain products such as whole wheat bread and crackers, whole-wheat bagels, cereals made from whole wheat or wheat bran, and muffins made with wheat bran will increase your fiber intake significantly. (Chapter 6 contains a lengthy discussion on a high-fiber diet because it is the major diet adjustment for an irritable bowel.) The second important point is that people with irritable bowel tend to tolerate breads, cereals, rice, and pasta well. In other words, these foods generally cause no or minimal irritable bowel symptoms. However, we caution you about what you put on starchy foods. For example, you may not tolerate a spicy tomato sauce with pasta, or a spicy curry dish over rice.

Many people believe that foods in this food group are fattening. For the most part this is just not true. It is what we put on these foods or how we prepare them that increases the calorie content. Opt to use small amounts or margarine or butter spread on bread and cream sauce over pasta, and know that frying rice adds fat to the grain. Enjoy a variety of foods from this food group, and for your health, choose lower fat choices (see "Healthy and Not So Healthy Choices" on page 30), and use spreads like butter, margarine, and cream cheese sparingly.

Some people try to increase their fiber intake by selecting bran muffins from a bakery or donut shop. These baked goods are

often are high in fat and sugar and hence calories. If you are concerned about weight gain, we caution you about doing this, as it
may result in an excessive calorie intake and increased weight.
We advise you to bake muffins (see our high-fiber, low-fat recipes
in appendix 3), buy a low-fat mix, or select low-fat varieties at
the bakery shop. Also, you can always choose other low-fat, low-
calorie, fiber-containing foods (see "Healthy Choices" below).

Healthy and Not So Healthy Choices

Healthy Choices	Not So Healthy Choices
whole-wheat or white bread	croissant
whole-wheat or white bagels	cheese bread
whole-wheat or white pita bread	cheese biscuits
low-fat whole-wheat crackers	garlic bread
steamed brown or white rice	cake with frosting
whole-wheat or white pasta or noodles	doughnuts
low-fat muffins	squares/sweets

What does a serving size look like?
- 1 slice of bread
- 1 ounce (30 g) of ready-to-eat-cereal
- 1/2 cup (120 ml) of cooked cereal, rice, or pasta
- 1/2 pita bread, 1/2 hamburger or hot dog bun, 1/2 bagel or
  1/2 English muffin
- 3–4 small crackers

Vegetable Group The vegetable group provides a lot of nutrition,
primarily vitamins A and C and folate, and minerals such as iron
and magnesium. Vegetables are low in fat, as long as they are prepared and eaten without added fat. Vegetables are also a good
source of fiber. Choosing a variety of vegetables provides you
with a variety of nutrients.

Legumes such as navy beans, pinto or kidney beans, and
chickpeas are in two food groups because they are a good source
of the nutrients found in both the vegetable group (fiber, vitamins, and minerals) and the meat group (protein). If you count
them as a vegetable serving, they do not count as a protein choice
at the same time.

For people who have gas and bloating, we often recommend

that particular vegetables be avoided or limited because of their gas-producing potential. (See page 67 for a list of gassy vegetables).

What does a serving look like?
- 1 cup (250 ml) of raw leafy vegetables
- 1/2 cup (120 ml) of other vegetables, cooked or chopped raw
- 3/4 cup (175 ml) of vegetable juice
- 1 small baked potato
- 1/2 cup (120 ml) of cooked legumes

Fruit Group Fruits and fruit juices have varied amounts of vitamins and minerals—in particular, vitamins A and C, potassium, and fiber. Like the vegetable group, choosing a variety of fruits is important to get the nutrition you need.

Like vegetables, certain fruits are particularly gas forming and may need to be limited or avoided in order to control gas and bloating symptoms (see page 68).

What does a serving size look like?
- 1 medium apple, orange, or banana
- 1/2 cup (120 ml) of chopped, cooked, or canned fruit
- 3/4 cup (175 ml) of fruit juice
- 1/2 cup (120 ml) of berries
- 1/4 cup (60 ml) of dried fruit

Milk, Cheese, and Yogurt Group Milk products provide calcium, protein, riboflavin, potassium, phosphorus, and vitamins A and D. In short, this food group is loaded with nutrition.

The group takes its name from the richest sources of calcium: milk, cheese, and yogurt. However, other dairy foods fit into this group, including cottage cheese, frozen yogurt, ice cream, puddings, and milk shakes.

Without milk products in your diet, it would be difficult to get enough calcium for your bone health.

The milk, cheese, and yogurt group is often an issue for people with digestive problems because they are frequently told to avoid milk products as a means to improve their gastrointestinal symptoms. This can lead to unnecessarily avoiding milk products. It's true that lactose or natural milk sugar may not be completely digested in some individuals and cause gas, bloating, and diarrhea. Lactose intolerance is not part of an irritable bowel, but in some people the symptoms are similar. On page 82 we can help you sort out whether you are lactose intolerant.

The milk, cheese, and yogurt group contains fat. But it is easy to reduce the fat you get from this food group by choosing lower fat items such as fat-free or 1% milk, fat-reduced cheese, and yogurt made with fat-reduced milk.

Some dairy products don't belong in this food group and should be limited because they are very high in fat and provide very few vitamins and minerals and little protein. Butter, cream, cream cheese, and sour cream belong with the fats, oils, and sweets group in the tip of the Pyramid, which should be used sparingly.

What does a serving size look like?
- 1 cup (250 ml) of milk, buttermilk, or yogurt
- 1 1/2 ounces (45 g) of natural cheese
- 2 ounces (60 g) of processed cheese
- 1/2 cup (120 ml) of frozen yogurt or 1 cup (250 ml) of cottage cheese = 1/2 serving
- 1/2 cup (120 ml) of ice cream = 1/3 serving

Meat, Poultry, Fish, Dry Beans, Eggs, and Nuts Group Meat, poultry, fish, and eggs provide protein, B vitamins, iron, and zinc. Dried beans and nuts provide similar nutrients but are also good sources of complex carbohydrates and fiber (and can also be counted in the vegetable group).

Dried beans and peas and nuts can worsen irritable bowel symptoms of abdominal gas and bloating, and therefore we recommend that people with these symptoms limit or avoid these foods (see page 68). Unfortunately, avoiding dried beans and peas, and nuts may be problematic for vegetarians and particularly vegans (who avoid meat, fish, poultry, eggs, and cheese). If you are a vegetarian and you want to control gas and bloating symptoms, we advise you to see a dietitian or nutrition professional to provide advice on how to get proper nutrition.

Meat can contain a significant amount of fat. You can keep the fat content of your diet lower by choosing leaner cuts of meat.

Examples of lean cuts of meat include round, loin, and sirloin beef, center loin, and tenderloin pork, ham, chicken or turkey without the skin.

What does a serving size look like?
- 2–3 ounces (60–90 g) of cooked lean meat, poultry, or fish (3 ounces of cooked meat is equal to the size of a deck of cards)
- 1 ounce of meat is equal to:
- 1/2 cup (120 ml) of cooked lentils, peas, or dry beans
- 1 egg
- 2 tablespoons (30 ml) of peanut butter
- 4 ounces (120 g) of tofu

Fats, Oils, and Sweets At the pyramid tip are fats, oils, and sweets. This is not an official food group, but is in the Food Guide Pyramid because we need some fats for our health. It's also there to acknowledge that fats, oils, and sweets are part of our normal diet. Still, these substances should be used sparingly. You may have noticed the dots and triangles throughout the rest of the Pyramid. They represent the fats or sugars either naturally occurring in other food groups (lactose—a sugar in milk—or the fat in cheese or meat) or added (sugar in ice cream or fat in a muffin recipe).

A few pointers for reducing fats and sugars in your diet:
- Choose lower-fat foods from the foods groups most often as we have suggested (see page 74).
- Use small amounts of fats and sugars when you cook or when you add to foods at the table—margarine, butter, gravy, salad dressing, sugar, and jam or syrup.
- Choose to eat high-sugar foods less often—sweet desserts, candy, and regular soft drinks. For desserts try angel food cake with unsweetened fruit, frozen yogurt, or fruit salad.

Snack-Attack Strategies
It's four in the afternoon, the time of day when you're most hungry. You're at the office, and you've got to have something to eat. What is going to satisfy your hunger and at the same time not increase your irritable bowel symptoms?

Contrary to what many people believe, snacking can be a part of a healthy diet. In fact, with an irritable bowel your digestive tract may tolerate smaller meals and in-between snacks better than it does a few hearty meals. Just make sure you choose healthy snacks and guard against overconsuming calories or fat.

Some snacks we know to be healthy are not well tolerated by people with an irritable bowel. For example, low-fat popcorn and raw vegetables should be avoided if you have problems with gas and bloating. These snacks are particularly troublesome when consumed on an empty stomach.

If you are concerned that snacking may lead to weight gain, especially if you cannot snack on raw vegetables, there are plenty of other low-calorie snacks. Look for low-fat starchy foods such as low-fat whole-wheat crackers or baby crackers. In addition to being low in calories and fat, they are well tolerated. Weight gain can also be avoided by keeping the size of your snack small, using the food label to know the size of one serving.

In general, starchy foods like breads, crackers, and cereal are well tolerated. The ideal starchy snack would contain whole wheat or wheat bran. Other foods such as milk, low-fat cheese or yogurt, fruit or fruit juice, or smooth peanut butter also tend to be well tolerated and may be combined with a whole-wheat starchy item.

Healthy Snacks If You Have an Irritable Bowel

- Low-fat wheat bran muffin (small to medium in size). Pass on the margarine or butter.
- Cereal and low-fat milk (best cereal choice is made with whole wheat). This is an excellent snack because it is low in fat (except granola-type cereals) and includes calcium-rich milk.
- Low-fat whole-wheat crackers, plain or with low-fat cheese or peanut butter. Eating only a few low-fat crackers can help you through a hungry period such as during meal preparation or the drive home after work.
- Low-fat yogurt—calcium rich and usually very well tolerated. Try various brands and flavors to decide which you like.
- Digestive, fruit-filled, or baby cookies. These snacks do not contain significant fiber, but they are well tolerated.
- Fresh fruit that you know you will tolerate (see page 68). Fruits generally tolerated are peeled apples, ripe pears,

peaches, and nectarines (when the skin and the fruit is soft), and bananas.

- Canned fruit. This is a well-tolerated snack. Choose the fruit packed in its own juice without sugar added.
- Pretzels and low-fat potato snacks.
- Whole-wheat toast. Use a very small amount of margarine or butter or try jam, low-fat cheese, or peanut butter. Make cinnamon toast by spreading on a small amount of margarine or butter and sprinkling with cinnamon sugar.
- Frozen yogurt. This is a good replacement for ice cream. Try the many different flavors and brands.
- Baked potato. This is a great choice for a warm snack. Try it plain or with a very small amount of margarine or butter. Another option is to add a small amount of grated cheddar or Parmesan cheese.
- Rice. Rice is well tolerated by people with an irritable bowel. Make a snack out of leftover plain rice with a small amount of margarine or butter or leftover rice casserole.
- Pudding. This calcium-rich choice is healthy as long as it is made with low-fat milk and with little added sugar. Rice and bread pudding are also possible choices.

Eating Out: Pleasure or Pain?

Eating out often presents a dilemma for people with digestive problems. Should you eat whatever you please and pay the consequences later? Or should you look over the menu carefully and pick items that will likely provoke the fewest, if any, irritable bowel symptoms? You may choose to "go for it" on some occasions and be cautious on others. Our advice is that if you eat out frequently (more than twice a week), you should choose menu items based on what you know you tolerate and like.

If you eat out infrequently, you may consider any discomfort you experience from eating foods that provoke irritable bowel symptoms well worth it. We don't disagree with this choice; we appreciate how you feel. Prepare yourself for symptoms. You won't damage your bowel, but you will make your symptoms worse. Managing symptoms is what this book is all about; therefore we cannot recommend that you eat any offending food on a frequent (daily) basis.

Most people choose their restaurants based on what they feel like eating and price. We suggest that you add another consideration—whether the menu includes items that are tolerated with minimal or no symptoms. It makes plenty of sense to choose a restaurant that offers menu items that will not trigger irritable bowel symptoms.

Tips for Pleasurable Healthy Meals When Eating Out

Don't be timid about asking your waiter about how a food is prepared, or that a menu item be prepared in a lean way if it is usually fried or served in a cream sauce. You may even inspire a change to more lean preparation techniques in the restaurant.

Choose tomato sauce rather than cream sauce. Tomato sauce usually has little added fat. If you have heartburn, ask that a small amount of cream sauce be added, or request it on the side.

Look for menu items that are prepared in lean ways—baked, broiled, char broiled, barbecued, stir-fried, poached, roasted, grilled, steamed, and braised. Healthy, hot meals that are generally well tolerated include:

- Char-broiled chicken or steak
- Grilled, broiled, or poached fish
- Baked or mashed potatoes, or steamed rice
- Cooked vegetables

Check the menu for sandwiches. Depending on the toppings, sandwiches are usually well tolerated if you have an irritable bowel. Request whole-wheat bread or a whole-wheat bagel to increase your fiber intake. If you have gas and bloating, skip sandwiches that are loaded with vegetables such as cucumber, lettuce, or tomato. Opt for a leaf or two of lettuce if you want to avoid irritable bowel symptoms.

Always request salad dressing on the side and use small amounts; however, salad may increase gas and bloating symptoms (see page 67).

For dessert choose frozen yogurt, sorbet, angel food cake, fruit salad (avoid citrus if you have heartburn, and melons or unpeeled apples if you have gas and bloating).

If eating at a fast-food restaurant, practice the tips for eating fast food found on page 76.

Chapter Five

Dietary Aggravators

Now that you understand how to adopt a healthy, balanced diet by following the Food Guide Pyramid, you are ready to look at how your diet—the foods you choose to eat and how you choose to eat them—may be provoking or aggravating your symptoms. Later in the chapter we provide strategies to remedy these diet-related causes.

Dietary aggravators of irritable bowel fit into three general categories:

1. Eating patterns. This refers to how you eat (when, where, how often, and how fast) and is closely related to your lifestyle, for example, whether you tend to eat breakfast or frequently eat at fast-food restaurants.

2. Symptom-provoking foods. This is what you eat. Many of our patients report an inability to tolerate foods without having symptoms. Fatty, gassy, or spicy foods are often singled out.

An important aspect to the symptom-provoking foods is how much you eat, whether you eat two or more symptom-provoking foods at once, or eat one or more at one meal and one or more at the next. All of these factors will have a bearing on whether you experience irritable bowel symptoms.

3. Insufficient fiber and water. All experts agree that a major aggravator of irritable bowel symptoms is insufficient fiber and water in the diet. We have seen this in our practice, too. By far the majority of patients referred to us do not have enough fiber or water in their diet.

Taking a Closer Look at the Symptom Aggravators

It is important for you to identify whether your particular symptoms are being caused by eating patterns, symptom-provoking foods, and/or insufficient amounts of fiber and water. This is one of the first steps in gaining control over an irritable bowel.

Eating Patterns

Some symptoms of irritable bowel are related to a person's lifestyle. Many of us find that we are too busy to take good care of our nutritional needs. As well, a busy lifestyle often means a stressful lifestyle. Irritable bowel symptoms are more pronounced when you are stressed (see chapter 7). Perhaps you can appreciate this from your own experience. When you feel stressed, this is the most important time to pay particular attention to your diet to make sure that your symptoms remain under control.

There are several common problems we see in patients in our clinic regarding eating patterns:

Eating too fast. Eating too quickly or on the run can result in indigestion. Indigestion refers to a discomfort after eating that may include feelings of discomfort in your stomach, bloating, reflux (stomach contents refluxing back up your esophagus), and heartburn. This results from eating quickly, so that your gastrointestinal tract does not have the ability to deal with the food in such a short time frame.

Eating fast food. A busy lifestyle, convenience, or just a liking for fast food may cause people with an irritable bowel to consume meals of pizzas, burgers, fries, or fried chicken from fast-food outlets. These foods tend to be hard to digest for people with irritable bowel. The foods are usually high in fat, which leads to indigestion, abdominal pain, and even diarrhea. There may also be other constituents in fast food such as preservatives that cause symptoms of an irritable bowel. Whether the cause is a high fat content or another constituent, generally fast foods are difficult to digest.

Skipping meals. Skipping meals or erratic eating habits (eating one meal per day or eating lots one day and little the next) provoke irritable bowel symptoms, particularly gas. Other symptoms are bloating, abdominal pain, and irregular bowel movements. Skipping meals may be related to a busy lifestyle. People may work through lunch, or parents busy with child care may not take the time to eat. Many women skip meals or eat lots one day and little the next as a weight control strategy. Unfortunately, it doesn't work. Plus it makes irritable bowel symptoms all the worse. Studies have shown that the skipped meal or the low-calorie day is more than compensated for by consuming more food at other times. Avoiding eating also triggers the body to store more energy as fat, thus defeating the "weight loss strategy."

Eating junk food. Junk foods are those foods that are high in calories but provide very few nutrients. They tend to be high in fat. Examples of junk foods are potato chips, nachos, cheezies, and chocolate bars. People with an irritable bowel who treat themselves at night to a snack of potato chips, nachos, or some other type of high-fat snack will likely find these hard to digest. High-fat snacks may result in indigestion, gas, diarrhea, and abdominal pain.

Overeating. The amount of food eaten is a critical point to consider. North Americans tend to overeat. Eating is at the center of most celebrations. We like to eat out and are doing this on an ever increasing basis. We have a tendency to overeat on these occasions likely because we consider them special. People with an irritable bowel do not tolerate eating in excess very well. With overeating comes indigestion, bloating, abdominal pain, and nausea, particularly if the meal is high in fat.

Your lifestyle can play an important role in provoking your irritable bowel symptoms. The most important point to realize is that the symptom-producing patterns or habits can be changed, and you are in control of that change. Later in this chapter we will review some general guidelines regarding eating patterns, which will help you keep your irritable bowel symptoms to a minimum.

Symptom-Provoking Foods

Many people with an irritable bowel do not digest fatty, gassy, or spicy foods well. These symptom-provoking foods and other poorly tolerated foods are called trigger foods. (See chapter 6 to find out which foods are fatty, gassy, and spicy.) These trigger foods may result in a variety of symptoms such as gas, bloating, diarrhea, and abdominal pain. In addition, there are many not so obvious trigger foods, for instance, food or drink that is high in caffeine. Caffeine causes frequent bowel movements in people who are prone to diarrhea, induces pain (from increased bowel contractions or spasms), and is a major cause of heartburn.

We noted earlier that how much you eat of a trigger food—whether you eat one or more of these foods at once or several throughout the day—will have a bearing on your experience of irritable bowel symptoms. Unfortunately, the effects of trigger foods can often be unpredictable, making it all the more perplexing for someone trying to sort out the mysteries of their symptoms.

Many patients come to us feeling very frustrated because they have not been able to pin down the problem foods. In fact, their frustration is so high that they have given up altogether trying to figure out what they can and cannot eat. Identifying trigger foods is indeed challenging. Some people have learned to avoid certain foods, but if other trigger foods remain in their diet, their symptoms will continue. Others attempt a high-fiber diet not knowing that fiber needs to be introduced gradually, that certain fibers make you feel gassy and don't help your bowel habit all that much, or that fiber does not work when you are not drinking enough water. Needless to say, these people arrive in our clinic feeling pretty lousy and frustrated. However, when they start to follow our advice, their symptoms improve dramatically.

A common lament goes like this: "The other night at a party I was concerned whether I could eat what was being offered. I was relieved when I saw that there was lasagna, Caesar salad, and rolls. The last time I had a lasagna I tolerated it fine, so I took some. I've had a problem with Caesar salad in the past, so I only had a very tiny amount. Not long after, I was never so sick! I left early and was up all night with gas, bloating, and diarrhea."

It's frustrating, but you may be able to tolerate a food at one time and not at another. Caesar salad (fatty and gassy) and spaghetti or lasagna (potentially gassy, spicy, and fatty) are examples of foods that you may tolerate only occasionally. Even your mother's turkey dinner (prone to overeating, potentially fatty, and possibly including a spicy stuffing) may represent a meal that you would tolerate only occasionally.

Usually if a situation is examined, a circumstance or two can be identified that contributed to the irritable bowel symptoms. For instance, for the person who attended the above party, we would have inquired whether she had any wine or other alcohol with her meal. Did she eat pâté or some other fatty appetizer that she forgot about? Was she stressed or excited? What did she have for lunch? What did she eat the previous day? Quite often when we examine the larger picture we can understand why symptoms flared up. However, there are instances when we cannot determine the cause of a patient's symptoms. You will experience situations like this. Don't be dismayed, though; they occur fewer and fewer times when you learn what foods trigger your symptoms, and the effective nutritional strategies to correct them.

In order for you to learn which foods are causing your symptoms, your diet and symptoms need to be examined in light of factors such as how much you ate of a potential trigger food and if you ate additional symptom-provoking foods with it, earlier in the day, or the day before. An important non-nutritional consideration is whether you are stressed. People with irritable bowel will always be more symptomatic when under stress. This is a general truth about the condition. Stress management is an important adjunct to nutritional management of irritable bowel symptoms. (Chapter 8 contains useful, practical guidelines on how to manage stress.)

The amount of potential trigger food a person can eat before experiencing symptoms depends on the particular food—and the person. Some foods, even if consumed in small amounts, provoke symptoms in most everyone with irritable bowel. Baked beans, pizza, and ice cream are common trigger foods. Some people with irritable bowel can tolerate small amounts of these and other trigger foods, but over a certain level of intake, symptoms occur. Coffee is another example of a trigger food that may not be tolerated at all, or just in small amounts, perhaps only one cup per day. It is clear, however, that people with irritable bowel will not tolerate excessive intakes of coffee—three or more mugs a day (6 to 8 oz. or 175–250 ml each)—without experiencing symptoms.

How often a trigger food is eaten has implications for irritable bowel symptoms. You may be able to tolerate certain foods occasionally if you don't eat them too often (or too much at once). Fatty, gassy, or spicy foods fall into this category. For example, some people prone to gas can eat a small side salad with a meal and tolerate this fine if they eat it once or possibly twice a week only. Also, some people can eat a fatty food such as a fast-food burger if they don't eat it more than once every week or two (and don't eat fatty French fries with it). Some patients tell us that they can tolerate the occasional bowl of moderately spicy chili fine, but they don't dare eat it two nights in a row (and they don't eat it with a gassy salad, or a side of refried beans).

Not So Obvious Trigger Ingredients

We mentioned earlier that there are constituents in foods that most people do not know can cause irritable bowel symptoms. The first is fructose. Fructose is the natural sugar found in fruits and berries. Fructose has been shown to increase abdominal distress in people with an irritable bowel. The symptoms are primarily gas, bloating, and diarrhea and appear to be related to bacteria in the large bowel digesting the natural sugar that was not completely absorbed in the small bowel. (See appendix 1 for information on the digestive process.) Apple juice, which is naturally high in fruit sugar, may be one of the causes of chronic diarrhea in children and adults. We see a fair number of people with diarrhea who are consuming six or more 8-ounce (250 ml) glasses of juice per day. When we ask them to decrease their intake to no more than one or two glasses daily, their diarrhea resolves.

The second food that may trigger your irritable bowel symptoms to be worse is regular soft drinks, which contain large amounts of table sugar. Large quantities of sugar are not well digested and result in diarrhea. We see people with diarrhea who have a 2-liter per day soft drink habit. The diarrhea is often further aggravated by the fact that the soft drink of choice tends to be a cola (dark) that contains caffeine. Again, when we advise these individuals to decrease their soft drink intake to no more than one or two 8-ounce glasses per day, their diarrhea resolves.

The third substance that can trigger irritable bowel symptoms is sorbitol, which may cause diarrhea. Sorbitol is found in a variety of fruits and plants and is used as a low-calorie sweetener. Sorbitol is not well digested, which makes it a good low-calorie sweetener. But this same property may produce symptoms of indigestion such as gas, bloating, diarrhea, and abdominal pain. Common foods containing significant amounts of sorbitol include peaches, apple juice, pears, sugarless gum, and dietetic jams and dietetic chocolate.

Another dietary constituent that may cause irritable bowel symptoms is olestra, a newer calorie-free fat substitute made from vegetable oils and sugar. Look for olestra's brand name Olean on the label of certain snack foods like potato chips and crackers. Olestra does not provide any calories because it is not digested or absorbed. Like sorbitol, this non-digestible characteristic may cause consumers of the product to experience digestive symptoms of gas, bloating, diarrhea, and abdominal pain. If you have these symptoms, check your diet for olestra content. You may need to reduce your intake of foods that contain this product.

Insufficient Amount of Fiber and Water?

Did you know that the average North American eats only half of the dietary fiber that they need? Instead of eating the recommended 20 to 35 grams of fiber daily, most people consume just 10 to 15 grams. For people with irritable bowel, a low fiber intake results in symptoms of constipation or diarrhea, or both, in an alternating fashion.

We wouldn't be surprised if you have tried a high-fiber diet in the past. You would be like the many patients who come to our clinic convinced that fiber will not work, or that they do not tolerate fiber. It makes perfect sense if you stopped a high-fiber diet when you found it didn't work or made you feel worse. However, you may have unknowingly fallen into the common pitfalls associated with trying a high-fiber diet without expert advice. Even some health care professionals, including physicians and dietitians, may have steered you wrong.

Not all health care professionals understand the important intricacies of a high-fiber diet for irritable bowel. This is one of the reasons that we, who specialize in gastroenterology, wrote this book. We know there is an unmet need for guidelines on how to manage an irritable bowel that are effective, based on clinical and experimental evidence, and practical.

Common Reasons a High-Fiber Diet Fails

Introducing a high-fiber diet too quickly. Fiber should be introduced gradually, over three to four weeks, and more slowly with some people.

Insufficient fiber intake. Some people think that if they eat whole-wheat bread, their diet is high in fiber. This is not so. Sometimes people eat lots of fiber some days, but little other days. In order to manage your symptoms effectively, a high-fiber intake is required daily.

The fibers that best regulate your bowel habit are not eaten in sufficient quantities. Wheat-based fibers such as breakfast cereals with wheat bran, whole-wheat bread, whole-wheat crackers, and wheat bran muffins are the most effective in regulating your bowel habit.

The required amount of water is not consumed. This is such a common mistake that we have come to expect it. We cannot make this point strongly enough: Eight 8-ounce (250 ml) glasses of water are required daily in order for the fiber to work. Some of our patients do not appreciate this on their first visit and do not drink enough water. When their symptoms improve only marginally, we again stress the importance of water consumption. On follow-up visits, the adequate water consumption, along with the high-fiber diet, has resulted in a regular bowel habit.

Some people do not like high-fiber foods. Fiber can be an acquired taste and may be brought into a diet over a period of time on a graduated basis. For example, starting with 60 percent whole-wheat bread, trying breakfast cereals made with whole wheat and combining this with a bran flake type cereal, and trying muffins make with whole-wheat flour. If you just don't think you can eat fiber-containing foods, we recommend a fiber supplement to control your symptoms.

Overcoming the Diet-Related Triggers of an Irritable Bowel

1. Change any eating patterns that are provoking your symptoms.

Eating too fast. Plan for allowing time to eat. Make this a priority. Once you have prepared a meal, sit and try to relax while you eat. Sit for a few minutes after you finish. If you must eat while working at your desk, take at least 10 to 15 minutes to eat your food.

Eating fast food. You will feel best if you limit the fast food in your diet. The maximum number of times you should eat fast food is once per week, and once every two weeks if you note that your symptoms are particularly bad with fast food. Fast-food restaurants offer healthy food choices such as a grilled chicken breast sandwich, baked potato topped with cheese and broccoli (may be gas forming) tossed salad (may be gas forming), and muffin. Try these for a change. Don't be misled into thinking all chicken and fish sandwiches are low in fat. Breaded and deep-fried chicken and fish sandwiches contain a lot of fat and therefore are likely not all that well tolerated. If you simply must have a burger, pass on the fries. French fries would substantially increase the fat content of your meal, making it harder to digest.

Skipping meals. In order to control your irritable bowel, it is important for you to eat three meals per day. You don't have to eat at precisely 7 A.M., noon, and 6 P.M., but you do need to eat something in the morning, afternoon, and evening. If you are concerned about weight gain, we are not suggesting that you eat large meals. Examples of balanced, very low calorie, nutritious meals that you are likely to tolerate include cereal, milk, and fruit in the morning, or a slice of toast and jam with a glass of juice; lunch could be a low-fat muffin and low-fat yogurt with a piece of fruit, or a sandwich on whole wheat filled with 1 ounce of a lean meat or cheese, and milk or yogurt; supper can be lean meat, fish, or chicken with rice or potato and vegetables, or pasta with a low-fat sauce (tomato, or a cream sauce made with milk and little fat), and some vegetables.

Keep in mind that eating small amounts throughout the day helps to curb your appetite. It also trains your body to burn off calories rather than storing them as fat, which is what happens if you eat only one meal per day.

Eating junk food. You don't need to give up junk food altogether. However, as with fast food, you will feel best if you keep your junk food intake to a minimum, perhaps once every one or two weeks. Also, you may need to decrease the amount of junk food you eat at once if you tend to eat large amounts (a large bag of potato chips or cheezies at a time). Try to cut this to less than half. Low-fat snack foods that you may tolerate better are pretzels, low-fat potato snacks, and whole wheat crackers. Sweeter low-fat snacks that you will likely tolerate are baby and digestive cookies, fig-, date-, or fruit-filled cookies, ginger snaps, breakfast cereal with milk (except cereals with nuts), granola bars without nuts, low-fat yogurt, and fruit canned in its own juice. (See page 33 for more on snacking and appendix 3 for recipe ideas.)

Overeating. Beware of those occasions that promote overeating, for example, family and holiday celebrations, office parties, eating out, or eating your favorite meal. Once you have had enough to eat, stop. Plan to eat what you could not, later. For example, have dessert a few hours after your meal or save some of your main course for a snack later on. You will enjoy and tolerate this much better. To help avoid overeating, drink water before you start a meal; this helps make you feel full and reduces your likelihood of eating too much.

2. Limit the symptom-provoking foods in your diet.

Trigger foods may be tolerated in small amounts, if eaten occasionally. However, we want to make it clear that it is important to follow your irritable bowel diet(s) closely for at least the first six weeks. (Chapter 6 presents the different irritable bowel diets.) If you don't follow the diet adjustments closely, you will not know whether the diet is effectively treating your symptoms. Once your symptoms are under control and you know how to treat them effectively, then you can experiment to see whether you tolerate certain trigger foods in small amounts, occasionally.

The Food Tolerance Test

Dietitians usually recommend that you test your tolerance to a suspect food in three steps:

- The first phase is to remove the food from your diet for a period of 2 to 6 weeks.
- After 2 to 6 weeks, try a small to moderate amount of the food in question, preferably with food you know that you tolerate, or by itself. Watch for symptoms you believe that the food causes. If you do not experience symptoms, it is likely that you tolerate the food, but you may need to test it another time to be sure.
- If you experience symptoms, put the food away for a week or more and try it again, in the same fashion—small amounts, with foods you tolerate, or by itself. If on the third try of a particular food you experience similar symptoms, then you do not tolerate the food. If you want to feel better, you should probably remove the food from your diet.

On occasions when you plan to enjoy a trigger food (after your symptoms are under control), eat a small to moderate sized portion and try not to have any other trigger foods with it or earlier in the day. For example, if you know that you are going to have a salad (gassy) with supper, don't eat trigger foods at noon. This will increase the likelihood that you will not tolerate the food that you are planning to enjoy at night. Strategies like this will keep your symptoms to a minimum.

If you plan to eat trigger foods over a period of time, such as over a holiday season, don't neglect consuming enough fiber and water, consistently. This should minimize the effects of trigger foods. So when you deviate from your diet, don't let it all go! You will want to feel well enough to enjoy the celebration.

3. Increase the amount of fiber in your diet.

Everyone who has irritable bowel will need an increased-fiber diet. Fiber is important for correcting your bowel habit whether you have constipation, diarrhea, or alternating constipation and diarrhea. The amount of fiber a person requires varies between 20 and 35 grams per day. The amount you need depends on the severity of your constipation or diarrhea. For example, if you have long-lasting constipation, and have difficulty moving your bowels once per week, your needs will be in the higher range, likely 25 to 35 grams per day. However, if you have constipation for 2 or 3 days, followed by loose stools for several days, your needs will likely fall into the 20 to 25 gram range. Chapter 6 contains guidelines on how to increase your fiber intake.

Food and Symptom Record

Now that you know the common nutrition-related causes of irritable bowel, it is time to discover the specific eating patterns, behaviors, and trigger foods that may be causing your symptoms. To do this we recommend that you use the Food and Symptom Record that starts on page 51.

For two weeks, please document the food you eat and the symptoms you experience. A two-week record is necessary to pick up patterns of symptoms and eating. What's more, symptoms may vary from week to week. Women in particular may notice that their symptoms change around their menstrual cycle. If this happens to you, we advise that you keep the record around this time. At the end of the two weeks, you should study your record to uncover the connections between the foods you ate or your eating patterns and the symptoms you experienced.

A food and symptom record is an important step in getting control over your symptoms. We highly recommend that you don't skip it. If is the most useful tool for looking at your diet and symptoms and determining the relationship between the two. If you don't keep a record, you may not appreciate that you have some symptom-provoking habits or eat some symptom-provoking foods. (It is like trying to drive with your eyes covered.)

How to Complete a Food and Symptom Record

We recommend that you record the six following irritable bowel symptoms that are treatable with diet, if and when you experience them over a two-week period:
- abdominal pain
- constipation

- diarrhea
- gas
- bloating
- heartburn (not an irritable bowel symptom but is associated with and irritable bowel)

Be sure to record both the foods you eat and the symptoms you experience. This is important because the specific diet adjustments that we recommend in chapter 6 are based on specific sets of symptoms. Each person who has an irritable bowel is unique. Symptoms, their type and severity, differ from person to person. If you do not have a problem with gas and bloating, or diarrhea, there is no need to follow the diet guidelines that are designed to control those symptoms.

To best track your meals, snacks, and symptoms:

- For greatest accuracy, make entries into the record throughout the day just after you eat or experience symptoms. If you are unable to do this, at least make your notes at the end of each day.
- Note all food and beverages consumed.
- Record the amount of food or beverage consumed. For example, 8 oz. skim milk or orange juice, a large potato, or one small chicken breast/skin removed.
- Write down how the food was prepared, for example, whether the chicken was fried or baked or you used 1 teaspoon of oil.
- In the section labeled "water," record the number of 8-oz. (250 ml) glasses of water you consume for that day.
- You will find your record easier to analyze if you write the foods in blue and the symptoms in red next to the foods you suspect provoked your symptoms.

How to Analyze Your Food and Symptom Record

Look at your eating patterns. Did you eat fast food, or junk food? Did you overeat? Did you skip any meals or eat lots one day and little the next? Do you remember eating quickly or on the run? Were you stressed? It may be easiest to answer each of these questions separately while analyzing your record for symptoms you may have experienced as a result. See page 54 for the symptoms that you may expect as a result of each eating pattern.

Analyze your record for any symptom-provoking foods. If you are unsure which foods are gassy, fatty, or spicy, see pages 67, 74, and 76 for tips on reducing fatty, gassy, and spicy foods. Remember, the amount of a trigger food is important as well as whether you ate one or more trigger foods at once. A combination of trigger foods may result in symptoms, but any one of them eaten alone may not. Whether you ate trigger foods throughout the day, or some the day before, is relevant and may make your symptoms worse. How much regular soft drink or juice did you drink daily?

Review your record for fiber and water content (see page 64 for fiber contents of common foods). Did you eat whole-wheat bread most of the time? Did you eat wheat bran cereals? How often? Did you choose whole-wheat crackers, or wheat bran muffins? How much water did you drink? How many 8-oz. glasses per day? On how many days, if any, did you drink eight 8-oz. (250 ml) glasses?

The food-symptom connections that you will identify through this record will tell you where to concentrate your dietary efforts in order to manage your irritable bowel symptoms. We recommend that you make a list of the foods and eating patterns that you singled out as causing your symptoms, as well as a separate list of the irritable bowel symptoms you experience.

ENLARGE THIS RECORD TO 200% ON YOUR COPIER

Food and Symptom Record

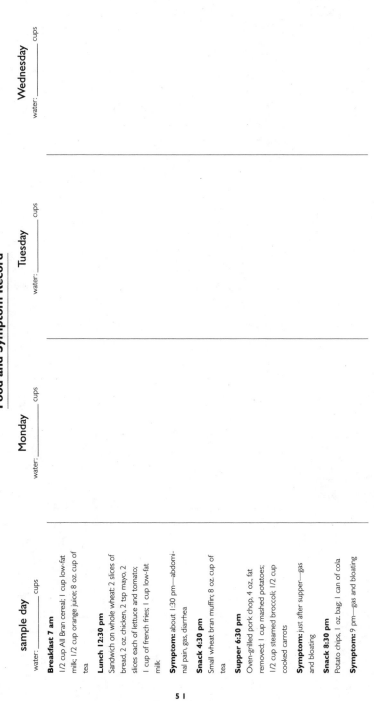

sample day	Monday	Tuesday	Wednesday
water: _____ cups	water: _____ cups	water: _____ cups	water: _____ cups

Breakfast 7 am
1/2 cup All Bran cereal; 1 cup low-fat milk; 1/2 cup orange juice; 8 oz. cup of tea

Lunch 12:30 pm
Sandwich on whole wheat: 2 slices of bread, 2 oz. chicken, 2 tsp mayo, 2 slices each of lettuce and tomato; 1 cup of french fries; 1 cup low-fat milk

Symptom: about 1:30 pm—abdominal pain, gas, diarrhea

Snack 4:30 pm
Small wheat bran muffin; 8 oz. cup of tea

Supper 6:30 pm
Oven-grilled pork chop, 4 oz, fat removed; 1 cup mashed potatoes; 1/2 cup steamed broccoli; 1/2 cup cooked carrots

Symptom: just after supper—gas and bloating

Snack 8:30 pm
Potato chips, 1 oz. bag; 1 can of cola

Symptom: 9 pm—gas and bloating

ENLARGE THIS RECORD TO 200% ON YOUR COPIER

Food and Symptom Record

Thursday
water: _____ cups

Friday
water: _____ cups

Saturday
water: _____ cups

Sunday
water: _____ cups

Chapter Six

Dietary Adjustments for Specific Symptoms

Before diving into this chapter, we strongly recommend that you first read chapters 4 and 5 if you haven't yet done so. They contain important tips for adopting a healthy diet as well as insights into how certain eating habits and food choices can provoke irritable bowel symptoms.

Diet is an essential component of treating an irritable bowel. And in our experience, nutrition management of irritable bowel symptoms is most often very effective.

In this chapter we offer specific diet adjustments and practical nutrition guidelines that have proven in our clinic and in research studies to be very effective at relieving irritable bowel symptoms. There's a lot to learn, so you may want to read this chapter more than once. It could prove difficult to digest (excuse the pun) in one reading.

The following table previews the recommended diet adjustments for the six most common symptoms associated with an irritable bowel. In the following pages we will explain each of these adjustments and show how they can work together if you experience more than one symptom at a time.

Matching Symptoms to Diet Adjustments

Irritable Bowel Symptom	Diet Adjustments
Abdominal Pain	High Fiber
	Low Gassy Foods
	Low Caffeine
	Low Fat
Constipation	High Fiber
	Low Caffeine
Diarrhea	High Fiber
	Low Caffeine
	Low Fat and Low Spice
Gas	Low Gassy Foods
	Low Caffeine
Bloating	Low Gassy Foods
	High Fiber
Heartburn*	Anti-Reflux

Matching Symptoms to Their Diet Adjustments

Abdominal pain stems from a number of other symptoms. It is associated with constipation or diarrhea, gases being trapped in the intestine, caffeine, or high-fat foods that are hard to digest. There are four potential diet adjustments based on the four potential nutrition-related causes.

Fiber treats the irregular bowel habit. If abdominal pain is due to gas, then a low gassy foods diet relieves discomfort caused by gas-producing foods. Caffeine may cause stomach pain, and therefore limiting caffeine will result in less pain. High-fat foods are hard to digest and may cause discomfort. Thus limiting fat in the diet will reduce pain resulting from digesting fatty foods.

The most important diet combination for treating the abdominal pain symptom is high-fiber and low gassy foods. In fact, this diet combination is recommend most in our clinic.

If you have spasms or intense shooting pain in your bowel, a high-fiber diet will benefit you; however, you will need to add fiber to your diet very gradually. You may also need to talk with you doctor about medication to treat this type of pain.

Constipation is primarily treated with a high-fiber diet. Fiber is recommended because it is a water-attracting substance and

---

*Technically, heartburn is not an irritable bowel symptom, but it is common with an irritable bowel.

therefore holds water in the stool, making it softer and easier to pass. When a person is constipated, fiber also speeds up the rate stools move through the large bowel.

Even though fiber can relieve constipation, not every high-fiber diet is appropriate for the person with an irritable bowel. A typical high-fiber diet needs to be modified to remove certain fibers that may be poorly tolerated. We often recommend removing certain fruits and vegetables, dried peas and beans, and nuts and seeds. These foods contain gas-producing fibers that result in more discomfort from gas than discomfort caused by constipation. We often recommend the high-fiber, low gassy food diet combination to treat constipation because irritable bowel patients who are constipated tend to have problems with gas and bloating. The high-fiber diet in this book is designed specifically for people with an irritable bowel (see page 58).

Diarrhea is thought to be caused by insufficient fiber in the diet; therefore a high-fiber diet is recommended. This surprises nearly all of our patients. Many people think that fiber causes their bowel movements to be loose. On the contrary, unless the diarrhea is due to an infection (intestinal flu) or inflammation (inflammatory bowel disease, I.B.D.) in your bowel, dietary fiber will help to form stool. This is not well known.

The reason fiber treats diarrhea is similar to why it treats constipation. Fiber, a water-attracting substance, holds excess water in a solid mass and forms the stool. Dietary fiber also slows the rate at which stools move through the intestine in people who have diarrhea.

Caffeine has been found to be a major cause of diarrhea for a significant number of our patients, so a low-caffeine diet is recommended to relieve diarrhea. Caffeine is a stimulant, and people who have diarrhea do not need their bowels to be stimulated.

Fatty or spicy foods can also cause diarrhea. You may have experienced this yourself on occasion. It is wise to limit fat and spice in your diet if you find that you experience diarrhea after eating spicy and fatty foods. This may mean reducing the amount of fat and spice you cook with and/or decreasing the number of times that you eat fatty of spicy foods. Chocolate, which contains caffeine and is high in fat, has also been linked to diarrhea and sometimes must be limited or avoided.

Gas is a common problem that causes bloating and abdominal pain, which occur when gas cannot be expelled. Nonetheless, producing and passing a lot of gas can make social situations uncomfortable. Therefore, a low gassy foods diet is appropriate when dealing with this symptom.

Gas also can come from swallowing air. When you eat quickly or gulp foods, you may draw air into your digestive tract. In addition, we have observed that some people have a lot of gas production when they drink coffee. We are uncertain of the reason for the gas production—perhaps the stimulant effects of caffeine—but the low caffeine guidelines may be helpful.

Bloating seems to be the most difficult symptom to treat. It may be due to constipation or eating gassy foods. It is treated with a high-fiber and low gassy foods diet. Often people who do not pass stools for two or more days feel bloated; a high-fiber diet will result in more frequent bowel motions. It also helps to remove from the diet gassy foods that contribute to the bloating. People who are prone to diarrhea may also experience bloating, but again, a high-fiber diet will help to regulate their bowel habit and minimize this bloating.

Heartburn is not a true symptom of irritable bowel, but it is associated with the condition. We include this symptom and the diet adjustment to correct it because in our experience, a significant number of people with irritable bowel suffer from heartburn. Coffee drinkers (caffeine) are also more likely to experience heartburn. Fortunately, heartburn is very amenable to diet adjustments.

Heartburn is caused by the underlying motility disorder associated with an irritable bowel. Because the gastrointestinal tract moves foods along in a disordered manner, the result is foods refluxing (going in reverse) from the stomach back up the esophagus. Stomach acids in the food cause the esophagus to feel like it is on fire, or burning. There are other reasons for heartburn, such as a hiatal hernia, which may cause you to reflux stomach contents, but the nutrition treatment is the same—an anti-reflux diet.

The anti-reflux diet removes foods that would otherwise cause the muscle in the bottom of the esophagus to weaken, which allows more foods to reflux and cause heartburn. The anti-reflux diet also removes acidic-type foods that people with reflux problems tend to tolerate poorly. When people with heartburn follow this diet, the results are usually dramatic. Even patients who require medication to get their symptoms under control can be weaned off drugs once they have been on an anti-reflux diet for several weeks.

Where Should You Start?

Very rarely does a person need to follow all six diet adjustments. You should choose your diet(s) based on your particular symptoms (see the table on page 54). Even then, you should probably start with just one diet adjustment. Three or four diet adjustments may benefit you; however, tackling that many diet adjustments at the same time is usually too much to manage.

We suggest starting with the high-fiber diet, since all people with an irritable bowel need between 20 and 35 grams of fiber in their diet daily. If gas and bloating are significant symptoms, then we suggest that you also try the low gassy foods diet at the outset. We suggest that you try both of these together because you will likely experience dramatic symptom relief. If initially you try the high-fiber diet alone, you may have less-effective results.

Your symptoms will tell you whether you need to introduce any other diet adjustments. The timing of diet introduction depends on two factors—the severity of a particular symptom and how many diet adjustments you feel that you can manage at the same time. For example, if you have become aware that caffeine is causing symptoms such as diarrhea or stomach pain, you may want to start the high-fiber diet (and low gassy foods diet if you have significant gas and bloating symptoms) and, at the same time, start to gradually reduce your caffeine intake. (For suggestions on how to cut caffeine consumption, see page 72.) Another example: If you are experiencing significant heartburn but little gas and bloating, you may want to start with the high-fiber and anti-reflux diets. Any further diet adjustments can be introduced later when you feel ready to try another adjustment.

Again, we recommend that you start with the high-fiber diet, accompanied by the low gassy foods diet if your symptoms of gas and bloating are significant. The next diet(s) that you introduce is up to you. We suggest that you base your decision on the type, number, and severity of symptoms you experience.

Be sure to try each diet adjustment for at least six weeks. This allows sufficient time for you to become adjusted to the diet and to evaluate its effectiveness.

The Diet Adjustments

The High-Fiber Diet: The Basic Factor

It takes 20 to 35 grams of fiber per day to regulate bowel movements. The amount you need depends on the severity of your constipation or diarrhea.

For a high-fiber diet to work, you will need to:

1. Eat the most effective type of fiber
2. Eat a sufficient amount of fiber
3. Eat a high-fiber diet every day
4. Drink plenty of water and other caffeine-free liquids daily

1.You need the most effective type of fiber. You may know that dietary fiber is found in whole-grain products, fruits and vegetables, and meat alternates such as nuts and dried peas and beans. These four different food groups contain different types of fiber.

Fiber is classified into two main types—soluble and insoluble. Most of these foods contain a mixture of fibers; however, some foods are known for the specific type of fiber they contain. For example, whole-wheat products and some vegetables like broccoli and carrots contain primarily insoluble fiber, while fruits, dried peas and beans, some vegetables, and oats are known for their soluble fiber content. Soluble fiber has a cholesterol-lowering effect in your body. This type of fiber also helps people with diabetes control their blood sugar.

Insoluble fiber, found in whole-grain wheat products, is the most effective in regulating your bowel habit. Examples are whole-wheat bread, whole-wheat crackers, wheat bran muffins, and breakfast cereals containing wheat bran. Insoluble fiber found primarily in whole-wheat products is the fiber of choice for the high-fiber diet.

As mentioned earlier, we often recommend avoiding certain fruits and vegetables, dried peas and beans, and nuts and seeds because the fibers in these foods produce excessive gas and worsen irritable bowel symptoms. Also, the fibers found in these foods are not as effective as wheat in regulating bowel habits.

(Guidelines on how to remove these foods from your diet are on page 47.)

It is very common for patients who come to our clinic to have tried a high-fiber diet in which they consumed lots of fiber from all sources. They report that they felt excessively gassy and bloated, and that there was little change in their bowel habit. They were focusing on fibers from certain fruits and vegetables, and dried beans. Once we advised them to focus on wheat-based fiber and avoid fiber that causes unreasonable amounts of gas production, their bowel habit improved, and their bloating and abdominal pain decreased.

The high-fiber diet recommended here focuses on wheat-based fibers. The fiber found in oatmeal and oat bran is not as effective as wheat in treating bowel habits. People with irritable bowel tolerate oatmeal and oat bran fine, but it will not help to regulate a person's bowel habit. Instead, wheat bran may be added to oatmeal (and other hot or cold cereals) to improve the amount and quality of fiber in order to regulate your bowel habit.

If you have a problem with gas and bloating and are on a high-fiber diet, you should not eat multigrain breads, crackers, or bagels because they may have sesame, poppy, flax, and sunflower seeds, which are likely to cause you to feel gassy. The best bread and crackers to buy if you want fiber but have a problem with gas and bloating is wheat bran, whole wheat, or wheat bread.

2. You need to eat a sufficient amount of fiber. A common mistake people make when they start a high-fiber diet is they simply eat whole-wheat bread and figure their diet is then high in fiber. Not so. There is more to a high-fiber diet than whole-wheat bread. Again, you will need to consume 20 to 35 grams of fiber per day. We will show you how to achieve this high-fiber intake with practical guidelines (see page 61).

People often ask if it is possible to eat too much fiber. Yes, it is. A fiber intake of more than 35 grams per day is too much for most people with an irritable bowel. If you consume more than this, you will likely experience discomfort in your belly and feel very bloated. Consuming more than 50 grams per day may decrease the absorption of some nutrients, such as iron, zinc, magnesium, and calcium.

3. You need to eat a high-fiber diet every day. A high-fiber diet needs to be followed seven days a week. Feel free to change some of your routine on weekends (sleep in, have brunch instead of breakfast and lunch), but you must eat that fiber.

4. Drink plenty of water and other caffeine-free liquids each day. This guideline is every bit as important as the first three. Fiber and water work very well together to regulate bowel movements, but neither works well by itself. As noted earlier, not getting enough water is likely the leading reason why high-fiber diets fail.

Drinking eight 8-ounce (250 ml) glasses of water each day can be a bit intimidating to some. However, like anything you embark on, once you get in the habit, it becomes much easier. It also helps to plan. Many patients in our clinic are successful when they drink two 8-ounce (250 ml) glasses of water with each meal. That means that six of the eight 8-ounce glasses of water daily are consumed at mealtimes alone. Drinking water with your meals also helps prevent overeating and facilitates the mixing of fiber and fluid in the digestive tract. Another option, whether you work outside the home or not, is to drink water throughout the day from a large covered container. Try to drink the equivalent of three 8-ounce glasses of water by lunch, and another three by supper. This makes six; you only need to drink two more.

If you take fiber in the form of a bulking agent such as Metamucil, you will be drinking one glass of water each time you take a serving. The manufacturer also recommends that you drink a second glass of water with each dose. If you take Metamucil twice daily, this represents half the water intake you need. However, if you divide your normal dose of Metamucil into three, you would be taking six 8-ounce glasses of water per day, or 75 percent of the water that you need.

Whatever scheme works for you, it is best to spread the water intake throughout the day and not leave it all to be consumed in the evening. We generally tell patients that 25 percent of the water requirement, or two 8-ounce glasses per day, may come from caffeine-free sources other than water, such as juice, milk, herbal tea, or noncola soft drinks. You may drink more of these liquids if you like, but count only two glasses for your daily water intake.

Making the Most of a High-Fiber Diet

For a high-fiber diet to be most effective, you should practice each of the following steps:

High-Fiber Guidelines

1. Choose wheat-based whole-grain products:
   - Whole-wheat bread
   - Wheat bran bread
   - Whole-wheat crackers
   - Wheat bran muffins
   - Whole-wheat cereal

2. Choose one concentrated source of fiber daily:*
   - A very high fiber cereal such as All Bran, 100% Bran, or Bran Buds with Psyllium
   - Natural Bran
   - Bulking Agent, such as Metamucil, Prodiem Plain, Norma-col, or Citrucel

3. Drink eight or more 8-ounce (250 ml) glasses of water daily.
   - Caffeine-free liquids such as juice, milk, herbal tea, and non-cola soft drink can be counted as two of the eight glasses of water per day.

These high-fiber guidelines are designed to regulate your bowel habit. Consequently, there is a major focus on whole-wheat and wheat bran products. To get the most fiber, check the fiber content on the food label and look for descriptors such as "high fiber," "good source," and "more fiber," or "added fiber," then select the item with the highest fiber content.

Fiber Content According to the Food Label

Description on Label	Meaning
High fiber	5 grams or more per serving
Good source	2.5 to 4.9 grams per serving
More or added fiber	at least 2.5 grams more per serving**

Also, check bread labels for the term "whole wheat." Breads with this term must be made from 100 percent whole-wheat flour. "Wheat bread," on the other hand, may contain some white

---

*It is important to introduce fiber gradually. See page 47.
**Compared to a standard serving size of the conventional food.

flour and some whole wheat flour. Check the ingredient list and buy the bread that contains the most whole-wheat flour.

Beyond choosing to eat whole-wheat products, we also recommend that you eat a concentrated source of fiber each day. (See page 63 for information about introducing a concentrated source of fiber into your diet.) This high-fiber source should be a part of your diet every day.

As the guidelines on page 63 note, there are several options for concentrated sources of fiber.

- Very high fiber cereals provide 10 or more grams of fiber in 1/2 cup (120 ml). They should only be substituted with a cereal of a similar fiber content.
- Natural bran, also called baker's bran, looks a bit like sawdust. In addition to being used in baking, it can be added to cereal and other foods to increase their fiber content.
- Bulking agents, such as Metamucil, Prodiem Plain, Normacol, and Citrucel, are made from natural plant fibers and are safe to take. They are not stimulant laxatives. Your bowel will not become dependent on them.

If you have never been a cereal eater, a bulking agent may suit you better than a very high fiber cereal. Maybe you would prefer to add natural bran to foods that you eat throughout the day. For variety, you may alternate your choice of a concentrated source of fiber from day to day. If you have primarily diarrhea bowel movements, such as four or more liquid stools per day, your best choice for a concentrated fiber source will be a bulking agent.

Gradually introducing a concentrated source of fiber is recommended because it might otherwise cause discomfort in the abdomen.

You may need to introduce the concentrated source of fiber more slowly than the above recommendations, especially if you have almost constant diarrhea or frequent and intense abdominal pain. If you have these symptoms, start with half of the amount suggested and increase by half of the amount in the times allotted. For example, start with 1/2 teaspoon (2 ml) of a bulking agent per day, and increase by 1/2 teaspoon (2 ml), instead of starting with 1 teaspoon (5 ml) daily, and increasing by 1 teaspoon (5 ml). Results may take longer, but you will tolerate the fiber better.

Introducing a Concentrated Source of Fiber

Very High Fiber Cereal: All Bran, 100% Bran, Bran Buds with Psyllium

Introduction: Start with 1/4 cup (60 ml) per day for 7 to 10 days, then increase to 1/2 cup (120 ml) daily. You may combine the very high fiber cereal with a lower-fiber cereal of your choice. For example, 1/2 cup of All Bran mixed with 1/2 cup of your favorite cereal.

Natural Bran

Introduction: Start with 2 tablespoons (30 ml) per day for 7 to 10 days, then increase to 4 tablespoons (60 ml) daily. Add to cereals, casseroles, stews, baked goods, whatever you like.

Bulking Agent: Metamucil, Normacol, Prodiem Plain, Citrucel

Introduction: Start with 1 rounded (not heaping, not level) teaspoon* (5 ml) each day for 7 days, then increase by adding another teaspoon at another time of day for 7 more days. You may need to add another teaspoon, preferably at a different time of day (1 teaspoon, 3 times a day), or double one dose (2 rounded teaspoons at one time, 1 teaspoon at another). You should not have to exceed a total of 4 rounded teaspoons per day.

*If you are using sugar-free Metamucil, I rounded teaspoon (5 ml) is recommended. If you are using regular Metamucil (contains sugar) use I level tablespoon (15 ml).

The final step in successfully adopting a high-fiber diet is to drink eight or more 8-ounce (250 ml) glasses of water each day. Skip this and the high-fiber diet will not work. Many people make great efforts to increase the fiber in their diet, but they do not consume enough water, which turns out to be the only reason that their bowel function does not improve satisfactorily. When they get the recommended amount of water, though, they get results: a regular bowel habit, and significant symptom relief.

It takes time for a high-fiber diet to start working, so it is wise to not expect results before the first two or three weeks. Your bowel is irritable! This means it may object to diet changes even if these changes will improve symptoms over the long run.

If you follow the high-fiber diet as advised—eating the recommended amount and type of fiber daily, and drinking eight 8-ounce (250 ml) glasses of water daily—and your bowel movements are better but not as regular as you would like, you may want to increase your concentrated source of fiber a bit more. For example, you may want to add another 1/4 to 1/2 cup (60 to 120 ml) of cereal in the afternoon, or take 1 to 2 rounded teaspoons (5 to 10 ml) of a bulking agent, or add 1 to 2 tablespoons (15 to 30 ml) of natural bran at a different time of day than when you ate your first concentrated source of fiber. You may need this extra concentrated source of fiber every other day only. As always, though, make sure that you have at least eight 8-ounce (250 ml) glasses of water daily.

Fiber Content of Selected Foods

Food, Portion Size	Dietary Fiber (g)
Grain Products	
whole-wheat bread, 1 slice (25 g)	1.7
wheat bran bread, 1 slice (25 g)	2.1
cracked wheat bread, 1 slice (25 g)	1.3
multigrain bread, 1 slice (25 g)	1.8
light rye bread, 1 slice (25 g)	1.6
wheat bran muffin, medium (4.4 × 5.7 cm diameter)	3.8
brown rice, long grain, cooked, 1/2 cup (120 ml)	1.5
white rice, long grain, cooked, 1/2 cup (120 ml)	0.4
whole-wheat noodles, cooked, 1/2 cup (120 ml)	2.3
white noodles, cooked, 1/2 cup (120 ml)	1.1
rolled oats, cooked, 1 cup (250 ml)	4.2
oat bran, cooked, 1 cup (250 ml)	5.7
cream of wheat, cooked, 1 cup (250 ml)	0.9
natural bran/baker's bran, raw, 2 Tbsp (30 ml)	3.0

Food, Portion Size	Dietary Fiber (g)
Legumes	
baked beans, 1/2 cup (120 ml)	9.9
dried peas, cooked, 1/2 cup (120 ml)	2.9
kidney beans, 1/2 cup (120 ml)	7.9
lentils, cooked, 1/2 cup (120 ml)	4.3
navy beans, cooked, 1/2 cup (120 ml)	6.3
Nuts	
almonds, dry roasted, unblanched, 10 nuts	1.6
peanuts, shelled, dry roasted, raw, 10 nuts	0.7
filberts, shelled, dried, unblanched, 10 nuts	0.9
peanut butter, chunky, 2 Tbsp (30 ml)	2.2
peanut butter, smooth, 2 Tbsp (30 ml)	1.8
Fruits	
apple, fresh with skin, 1 medium	2.6
apple, fresh without skin, 1 medium	2.4
applesauce, 1/2 cup (120 ml)	1.5
apricots, dried, 5 halves, uncooked	1.4
apricots, fresh, 3 whole	2.0
banana, 1 medium	2.0
blueberries, fresh, 1/2 cup (120 ml)	2.0
cantaloupe, 1/4 whole	0.9
cherries, sweet, 10	0.7
dates, 3	2.0
grapefruit, 1/2	0.8
grapes with skin, 1 cup (250 ml)	0.8
orange, 1 medium	2.4
papaya, 1 medium	5.3
peach, fresh, 1 medium with skin	1.6
pear, fresh, 1 medium with skin	5.0
pineapple, 1/2 cup (120 ml)	0.9
plums, 5 damson	5.3
prunes, 3	1.8
raisins, 1/4 cup (60 ml)	2.5
raspberries, 1/2 cup (120 ml)	3.0
strawberries, 1 cup (250 ml)	3.0
rhubarb, cooked, 1/2 cup (120 ml)	1.7

Food, Portion Size	Dietary Fiber (g)
Vegetables	
asparagus, cooked, 4 spears	1
bean sprouts (Mung), raw, 1/2 cup (120 ml)	0.6
beans, green or yellow, cooked, 1/2 cup (120 ml)	1.5
beans, lima, cooked, 1/2 cup (120 ml)	4.3
broccoli, cooked, 1/2 cup (120 ml)	1.9
brussels sprouts, cooked, 1/2 cup (120 ml)	3.4
cabbage, cooked, 1/2 cup (120 ml)	1.3
carrots, cooked, 1/2 cup (120 ml)	2.1
carrots, raw, 1 medium	2
cauliflower, cooked, 1/2 cup (120 ml)	1
celery, raw, diced, 1/2 cup (120 ml)	0.9
corn, cooked, 1/2 cup (120 ml)	3
corn, 1 ear (30 cm)	6.6
onions, raw, diced, 1/2 cup (120 ml)	1
parsnips, cooked, 1/2 cup (120 ml)	3.1
peas, green, cooked, 1/2 cup (120 ml)	3.6
potatoes, baked, 1 medium w/skin	4.5
potatoes, boiled, 1 medium w/skin	4
potatoes, mashed, 1/2 cup (120 ml)	2.5
spinach, cooked, 1/2 cup (120 ml)	2.1
spinach, raw, 1 cup (250 ml)	1.5
squash, winter, all varieties, baked, 1/2 cup (120 ml)	2.9
summer, all varieties, boiled, 1/2 cup (120 ml)	1.5
sweet potato, baked in skin, 1/2 medium	1.7
sweet potato, boiled without skin, 1/2 medium	1.8
sweet potato, candied, 1 piece	2.3
tomato, raw, 1 medium	1.5
turnip, cooked, 1/2 cup (120 ml)	2.3

Source: Health Canada. Health Protection Branch. Canadian Nutrient File. Version 1997. Numbers rounded to the nearest one-tenth gram.

The Low Gassy Foods Diet: Go Further on Less Gas

A high-fiber diet is often teamed with a low gassy foods diet to ease a number of irritable bowel symptoms. Reducing the amount of gassy foods in your diet will help to treat the symptoms of abdominal pain, gas, and bloating.

Certain foods are gassy because they contain carbohydrates, a form of sugar, which are not completely digested in the small bowel (the section of bowel connected to the stomach; see page 145 for information on how the gut works). When these sugars get to the large bowel, lots of bacteria digest them and, in the process, produce gasses. This is what makes you feel gassy, bloated, and in pain.

Certain fruits and vegetables and dried beans and peas may make you feel particularly gassy and bloated. This is because these foods contain the carbohydrates that are usually not totally broken down in the small bowel.

It is common for bloating to become worse as the day progresses. Some people say they practically need a size larger clothing by the evening! Fortunately, cutting down on gassy foods will bring relief to your bloating-type symptoms.

Low Gassy Foods Guidelines

1. Pay attention to how you are eating.
   - Try to avoid gulping foods or eating quickly, as this may increase gas production.
   - Try not to skip meals. This allows the gastrointestinal tract to fill with air.
   - Avoid chewing gum or sucking on hard candy, which introduces lots of air into the gastrointestinal tract.
   - Avoid using a straw to drink liquids. More gases are swallowed using straws.

2. Pay attention to what you are eating. Certain foods are gas forming. Avoid (for at least the 6-week trial period):
   - All raw vegetables, including salads.
   - The following vegetables, even if they are cooked:

broccoli	cauliflower
brussels sprouts	cucumber
cabbage	corn

kohlrabi	rutabaga
leeks	sauerkraut
onion	scallions
red/green pepper	shallots
pimentos	turnip
radish	

- Dried peas, beans, and lentils such as:

black-eyed peas	navy beans
kidney beans	split peas
lima beans	lentils

- The following fruits:

unpeeled apples	honeydew melon
avocados	prunes
cantaloupe	watermelon

- Miscellaneous foods:

beer	seeds
hard-boiled eggs	soft drinks
nuts	wheat germ
popcorn	

3. Choose the following foods:
   - Vegetables to choose, cooked:

asparagus	potato
beets	sweet potato
carrots	spinach
green beans	squash
yellow beans	pumpkin
green peas	zucchini
mushrooms	

   - Fruits to choose:

canned fruit	nectarine
peeled apples	orange
soft, ripe banana	peach
grapefruit	pear
kiwi	

In looking over the low gassy foods guidelines, you likely noticed the number of fruits, vegetables, and other foods that should be limited or avoided. Although these foods are otherwise healthy, they are not tolerated very well by people with an irritable bowel who have gas and bloating as significant symptoms.

Fortunately, there are nutritious fruits and vegetables that are known to be less gassy (see guideline 3 on page 68). To minimize their gas-producing qualities, vegetables should be cooked and fruit canned or eaten ripe (when the fruit and skin is soft). Some people report that bananas cause stomach pain. If you find that any of the suggested fruits and vegetables bother you, it would be wise to avoid them.

Because the low gassy foods diet restricts many fruits and vegetables, the produce you do eat should provide optimum nutrition. Some of the most important nutrients to obtain are beta carotene (or vitamin A), vitamin C, and folate.

Carotenoids, particularly beta carotene, which changes into vitamin A, perform many functions in your overall health. Plus, as an antioxidant, vitamin A may offer protection from some diseases and aspects of aging. Vitamin C is another antioxidant vitamin that protects the body much the same way as vitamin A. Among many other responsibilities, vitamin C helps form the connective tissue that holds the many structures of the body together. It also keeps capillaries and gums healthy and helps the body to absorb iron from plant sources.

Folate is particularly important for all women of childbearing age. Pregnant women who do not get enough folic acid (folate), especially during the first trimester, have a greater risk of delivering a baby with neural tube defects such as spina bifida. The U.S. Food and Drug Administration has made it mandatory that enriched flour be fortified with folate as of January 1998. This means that the baked products and pasta that you buy (with "enriched flour" written on the label) or enriched flour you use in baking will be fortified with folate. If you eat 6 servings of enriched grain products daily, you will have 80 percent of the folate that you require.

The following foods are generally well tolerated by people with irritable bowel. Try to choose these foods as often as you can. Remember, the vegetables will need to be cooked.

Well-Tolerated Nutrient Powerhouses

Vitamin A	Vitamin C	Folate
carrots	orange/orange juice	orange/orange juice
pumpkin	grapefruit/grapefruit juice	spinach
sweet potato	tomato/tomato juice	asparagus
spinach	baked potato with the skin	
winter squash	spinach	

As you can see, some foods are high in more than one nutrient. For example, orange juice is high in vitamin C and folate; tomatoes are high in vitamin A and C; and spinach is high in all three nutrients.

If you are following a low gassy foods diet, there are circumstances when a multivitamin/mineral supplement is suggested:

- If you do not like or regularly eat the foods that contain significant amounts of vitamins A and C and folate.
- If you are also following an anti-reflux diet. The anti-reflux diet removes tomato and citrus fruits from your diet (see page 77).

If you feel less gassy and bloated at the end of the usual 6-week trial period, we suggest that you add in the foods that you missed the most—in small amounts, occasionally. For example, if you miss cauliflower, try a small to moderate amount at a meal (see page 47 about tolerating foods). If you really missed eating salads, try a small side salad with foods that you know you tolerate. Remember, though, certain foods may always provoke symptoms no matter how little you eat or how infrequently.

It's best to keep your intake of any gassy foods to small to moderate size servings, two or three times a week. If you reintroduce gassy foods and eat them as often as you previously did, then you will likely feel as you did before you started the low gassy foods diet.

If the low gassy foods diet does not significantly relieve the gas and bloating in 6 weeks, the restrictions are not working, and you should discontinue the diet.

By choice or mistake, you are bound to eat foods that will make your symptoms worse. Patients often worry that they are causing damage to the bowel by eating offending foods, but this is not the case. As we've said before, no bowel damage will result from eating trigger foods, only increased symptoms. This is why we can comfortably say that it is your choice to eat trigger foods.

The Low-Caffeine Diet:
Who Needs Jumper Cables?

The low-caffeine diet is significant for people with irritable bowel because caffeine is a stimulant to the muscles in the digestive tract. You know how caffeine stimulants your brain—it wakes you up. It has a similar effect on the digestive tract. Caffeine can cause diarrhea, heartburn, stomach pain, and, in some cases, gas. You don't need to have an irritable bowel to have a problem tolerating coffee. However, an irritable bowel is particularly susceptible to the effects of caffeine.

Caffeine has been part of our diet for centuries. It is found naturally in plants such as coffee, tea, and cocoa and is added to soft drinks and nonprescription medications. Caffeine behaves like a natural "diuretic," which means that it causes fluids to move quickly through the kidneys. Interestingly, this effect may make it more difficult for bran to combine with water to form a soft stool.

The major source of caffeine in our diet is coffee, with colas (dark soft drinks) running a close second. Drip coffee—the coffee sold in most coffee shops and restaurants, and often the coffee of choice at home—contains the most caffeine (see page 73 for the caffeine content of selected beverages). Not surprisingly, decaffeinated coffee is the lowest in caffeine. Even so, decaffeinated coffee can cause just as much stomach acid secretion as regular brew. Therefore, if you experience stomach pain or heartburn as a result of drinking coffee, you may find that even decaf brings no relief. If so, it is best to remove all coffee from your diet.

For most adults, the caffeine in two 6-ounce mugs (175 ml) of coffee per day generally causes no harmful effects. If you can drink this much without diarrhea, heartburn, and stomach pain, great. But don't drink any more. Many people, though, find that even less coffee causes their irritable bowel symptoms to be worse. If caffeine seems to trigger your symptoms, we advise that you remove coffee from your diet. Giving up or reducing your caffeine intake is a challenge, so we have compiled a list of strategies to help you.

Cutting the Caffeine

Caffeine is a drug. We can become dependent on it. Therefore, giving it up or significantly limiting the caffeine in our diet is easier said than done. However, the benefits of eliminating or significantly decreasing the caffeine in your diet will be well worth the effort especially if you are prone to diarrhea, heartburn, or stomach pain.

Coffee

1. You may be one of those people who has more success when you give up something all at once. If this is your style, great; your digestive tract will like you. If you go cold turkey, you may experience headaches and tiredness initially, but this disappears in 7 to 10 days. If you prefer a more gradual approach...

2. You might want to start by trying to stop drinking coffee after a certain hour in the day—3 P.M., for example. Once you have successfully done this, try stopping at noon, and work so that you are consuming only one or two cups of coffee per day. If you are still experiencing symptoms, we suggest that you remove coffee from your diet. You may need more steps in the plan, depending on how much coffee you drink.

3. Mix your regular coffee with decaffeinated, initially drinking the same number of cups per day. Once you have adjusted to half regular/half decaf, you may gradually work on decreasing both the amount of regular coffee as well as the number of cups of coffee in your diet daily.

4. Mix your coffee with equal amounts of milk while keeping the size of your cup the same. This has the added bonus of providing some milk products in your diet. After drinking half coffee/half milk for a while, you can then work on decreasing the number of cups of coffee that you drink daily.

5. Switch to instant coffee, which has half the caffeine content of filter drip. The two are not equal in flavor, but remember that you are trying to give up coffee. After you switch most of your coffee intake to instant, reduce the number of cups you have each day.

6. Replace your coffee with herbal tea. Herbal tea is caffeine free and is much like consuming water. The bonus with herbal tea is that it contributes to your caffeine-free liquid intake. Plus, you still get to enjoy a hot beverage. There are many herbal teas on the market, so you may need to experiment with flavors before you find the one(s) you like.

Cola

1. Smooth the switch to a noncola soft drink by first choosing decaffeinated colas or light-colored soft drinks. If one of your irritable bowel symptoms is lots of gas production, switching to a noncola soft drink will not help relieve this symptom. You will be better off removing or severely reducing the soft drinks in your diet no matter what the flavor.

2. Replace some of your cola intake with ice water, which is very thirst quenching and counts toward your daily caffeine-free liquid intake. You might even use some juices to satisfy your thirst. This is a very healthy choice. Keep in mind that excessive juice intake (more than three 8-ounce glasses per day) can cause loose bowel movements.

Caffeine Content of Selected Beverages

Sources of Caffeine	Caffeine (mg)
Coffee (per 6 oz. or 175 ml)	
Automatic percolated	72–144
Filter drip	108–180
Instant regular	60–90
Instant decaffeinated	<6
Tea (per 6 oz. or 175 ml)	
Weak	18–24
Strong	78–108
Cola soft drinks (12 oz. or 335 ml), 1 can	18–64

Adapted from *Caffeine and You (It's Your Health)*, Health Canada, January 20, 1993. With permission of the Minister of Public Works and Government Services Canada, 1997.

The Low-Fat Diet: Lose the Fat

The low-fat diet will help reduce symptoms of abdominal pain and diarrhea. But how low does a low-fat diet need to go? The good news here is that you do not need to eat any less fat than is recommended for the general population. The Dietary Guidelines for Americans recommend that fat represent 30 percent or less of your daily calorie intake, with no more than 10 percent of the total intake coming in the form of saturated fat (fat from animal sources such as dairy products, beef, chicken, pork, eggs; and hydrogenated fats). Your bowel does not recognize the difference between types of fat (saturated versus unsaturated), but your heart and blood vessels do. Therefore, this low-fat diet is low in total and saturated fat.

Beyond how much fat is consumed over a period of days, it is important to limit the amount of fat in a particular meal or snack. Fat is better tolerated when eaten in small amounts throughout the day. Fat is hard to digest, and large amounts can cause the bowel to be irritable.

Low-Fat Guidelines

1. Limit your fat intake from visible fats:
   - Lightly spread margarine or butter (1 teaspoon or less)
   - Choose light margarine
   - Use jam or jelly rather than margarine or butter
   - Choose low-fat or fat-free mayonnaise and salad dressings
   - Choose low-fat or fat-free sour cream

2. Choose low-fat dairy products:
   - Drink skim or 1% milk
   - Choose fat-reduced yogurt
   - Choose fat-reduced cheese such as low-fat cheese that contains <20% milk fat or skim milk cheese that contains <7% milk fat
   - Choose frozen yogurt, low-fat ice cream, or frozen ice milk

3. Choose lean meats and use low-fat cooking methods.
   - Lean cuts of beef—round, sirloin, blade, lean ground, filet, stew meat

- Lean cuts of chicken—skinless chicken breasts; other cuts, skin and fat removed before cooking
- Lean cuts of pork—tenderloin; loin chops; and ham with fat removed before eating
- Lean cooking methods—barbecuing, baking, broiling, roasting, stewing, steaming, braising

4. Choose lower-fat sandwich fillings.
   - Lean fillings—sliced beef, chicken, ham, pastrami, turkey, and low-fat cheese
   - Use low-fat mayonnaise in egg, tuna, or salmon salad.
   - Pass on margarine or butter for the bread; choose low-fat mayonnaise, or a variety of mustards.

5. Watch out for hidden fats.
   - Make low-fat or reduced-fat muffins, biscuits, pancakes, and waffles rather than buying their higher-fat versions from the bakery or grocery store. (See appendis 3 for high-fiber, low-fat recipes.)
   - Buy low-fat bakery goods.
   - Choose crackers with no more than 5 grams of fat per serving. Even whole-wheat crackers contain hidden fat.
   - Avoid crackers made with tropical oils such as coconut, palm, or palm kernel. These are highly saturated, and bad for your heart.

The greatest source of dietary fat comes from fats that we spread on or add to foods, such as margarine, butter, mayonnaise, salad dressings, and oil. These fats are called "visible fats" because we can see them. We can also usually control how much visible fat we consume. For this reason, making changes here can significantly reduce the fat content of your diet.

Another strategy to significantly reduce your fat intake is to choose low-fat dairy products. It is important that we consume dairy products, but we are recognizing that it is equally important to consume the lower-fat milk products. All grocery stores carry lower-fat milk, cheese, and yogurt. In fact, the selection has never been better. You will find a variety of spreadable and hard cheeses, yogurt, and frozen yogurts on the shelf. Experiment with a few that you have never tried. We believe that you will find cheeses and yogurts that you enjoy just as much as the full fat varieties.

Choosing lean cuts of meat and preparing them in low-fat methods can also make a difference in the fat content of your diet. Try to limit your protein intake to the recommended amount: 5 to 7 ounces (150 to 210 g) per day.

North Americans are known for their fondness for sandwiches: subs, clubs, burgers, heros, old standbys of sliced meats and cheese. Cut the fat in your diet by choosing lower-fat sandwich fillings and watching the amount of spreadable fat (butter, margarine, and mayonnaise) you put on them.

Finally, as you follow the low-fat diet for an irritable bowel, watch out for the "hidden fats" in foods. Hidden fats are fats that you don't necessarily see, but they are present in significant amounts in certain foods such as crackers, muffins, biscuits, and other baked items. Choose low-fat crackers and muffins. (See appendix 3 for high-fiber, low-fat recipes).

The Low-Spice Diet:
Who Needs Spice in Their Life?

The question of "spicy foods or not?" is common among people with an irritable bowel. Everyone tolerates spicy foods differently—irritable bowel or not. However, we have found that those with an irritable bowel may not tolerate foods that contain these spices:

chili powder	curry
hot chili peppers	ginger
garlic	spicy BBQ sauce
hot sauce	

You may tolerate these spices in small amounts, but if they are prominent in a dish, you may experience gas, bloating, and diarrhea. We cannot provide exact amounts that you will tolerate. It is up to you to experiment a bit with spices if you are not already certain what types and amount you can tolerate. If you choose to experiment, we suggest that you start with smaller amounts (see page 47 for testing your tolerance to foods).

Some people mistakenly believe that herbs are difficult to digest. On the contrary, herbs such as basil, oregano, thyme, and rosemary are usually well tolerated if you have an irritable bowel. It's usually the other foods in a dish that cause symptoms. For example, lasagna, which can be very high in fat depending on the type and amount of meat and cheese used, can also contain lots of garlic. The high fat content, garlic, or tomato sauce (particularly for people who have heartburn) may cause a person to have abdominal pain, diarrhea, or heartburn. To add flavor to your diet, you may want to experiment with herbs.

The Anti-Reflux Diet:
Moving in the Right Direction

You only need to be concerned with the anti-reflux diet if you have heartburn. Officially, heartburn is not a symptom of irritable bowel, but it is associated with it.

Heartburn is the pain you get in your upper chest after acidic stomach contents back up (reflux) into your esophagus. Your esophagus is the hollow tube that food travels through to your stomach. (See page 145 for more information on how the gut works.)

Normally, stomach contents leave your stomach and enter your small bowel, but with heartburn they travel back into your esophagus, in the wrong direction. Your stomach and small bowel are designed to handle an acidic environment, but your esophagus is not; hence you get that burning sensation when acids make contact with the lining of your esophagus (just like your skin would burn if touched by acid).

Heartburn is a fairly common problem in North America. It affects an estimated 30 percent of all adults—7 percent on a daily basis. Heartburn occurs for a number of reasons, though not all people who have heartburn have an irritable bowel. Sometimes the refluxing of stomach contents is easier because of a hiatal hernia, which is part of the upper stomach protruding above the diaphragm. However, many people who have a hiatal hernia do not have symptoms of heartburn. Another possible cause of heartburn is a weak lower esophageal sphincter (LES). This muscle sits at the bottom of the esophagus where the esophagus meets the stomach. The LES opens when we swallow and closes right after the food passes into the stomach. If it is weak, though, the muscle does not close effectively, and acidic stomach contents can reflux back up the esophagus and cause heartburn.

Anti-Reflux Guidelines

1. Avoid the following foods, which are likely causes of heart-burn:
- caffeine—particularly coffee, strong tea, and cola beverages
- citrus fruits—orange, grapefruit, lemon, and lime
- tomato—in any form
- fatty foods, including fried foods; fatty meats such as bologna, salami, and regular hamburger; and potato chips, peanuts, ice cream, and rich desserts

2. Avoid other trigger foods, including:
- alcohol
- peppermint
- chocolate
- spicy foods (see page 76)

3. Wait at least 2 hours after eating before lying down; a bedtime snack may not be tolerated.

4. Try eating smaller meals.
- plan to snack midmorning or midafternoon if you get hungry.

5. Drink most fluids between meals.

6. You may need to limit your intake of gas-forming foods such as:

broccoli	raw vegetables, including
brussels sprouts	salads
cabbage	dried peas and beans
cauliflower	soybeans
corn	unpeeled apples
green peppers	cantaloupe
onion	honeydew and watermelon
turnip	

The key to following the anti-reflux guidelines is to remove food triggers that cause the LES to weaken, and to make some general lifestyle changes that minimize reflux.

The first order of dietary treatment is to remove from your diet the notorious trigger foods for heartburn:

caffeine	tomato
citrus fruits	fatty foods

If you are a coffee lover, you may want to go decaffeinated. However, decaf does trigger acid secretion just like regular coffee, therefore, it may not provide relief from heartburn. Your best bet is to remove coffee from your diet (see page 72 for tips), or limit it to one cup per day if you feel that you cannot give it up. That one cup may still cause heartburn, but like all potential trigger foods, it is your choice to keep it in your diet.

Citrus fruits and their juices are not well tolerated in people who have heartburn. You may want to try other fruit juices such as apple or cranberry, which are sometimes perceived as being less acidic. A number of patients tell us that they cannot drink juice of any kind without getting heartburn. Before removing all juices from your diet, we recommend that you try non-citrus juices that are fortified with vitamin C.

Tomato is a major cause of heartburn. Unfortunately, it does not matter in what form you consume it—soup, salad, sandwich, or sauce. The best advice is to avoid tomatoes in all forms.

Fatty foods often trigger heartburn in susceptible people. By fatty foods we mean fried foods such as fried chicken, fried hamburgers, fried steak, fried fish (especially in batter), or French fries. Other fatty foods are fatty meats such as salami, pepperoni, regular hamburger, bologna; high-fat snacks such as potato chips, tortilla chips, and peanuts; and rich desserts and ice cream. Pasta made with a cream sauce, or casseroles made with a cream or cheese sauce, may also be high in fat and cause heartburn.

Besides the main heartburn triggers, a few foods are what we call secondary triggers of heartburn. These substances may not trigger heartburn in all people if consumed in small amounts. After 6 weeks, you may want to check your tolerance to these substances (see page 47 for more information on testing your tolerance to foods).

Your chance of heartburn can also be lowered by waiting at least 2 hours after eating before you lie down. Stomach contents are more likely to back up your esophagus (reflux) when you lie down. When people wake up with heartburn in the middle of the night, it's usually because they ate an evening snack. If you are accustomed to a bedtime snack, you will need to eat this 2 or more hours earlier and make it light, such as a small bowl of cereal or a slice of toast. You may even find that you can't eat an evening snack at all without waking up with heartburn. In this case it is best to avoid snacking in the evening. Another strategy for reducing heartburn and acid reflux at night is to sleep with the head of the bed elevated on blocks that are about 6 inches (15 cm) high.

Sometimes people feel better and have less heartburn if they eat small meals and snack if they get hungry. You are more likely to reflux a large meal because an overdistended stomach puts pressure on the food to move upward. Drinking a lot of fluid (more than two 8-ounce or 250 ml glasses) with meals may cause reflux. Try to keep your liquid intake with meals or snacks equal to or less than this amount.

Finally, some gassy foods may reflux into your esophagus, though this is not common. In the interest of thoroughness, we have included this possibility. Should you find that a variety of gassy vegetable and fruits cause you to have heartburn, see page 67 for guidelines about low gassy foods and advice on meeting your nutritional requirements.

More Diet Adjustments

Alcohol: More Than an Appetite Stimulant

We are often asked about the effects of alcohol on an irritable bowel. Alcohol is a stimulant to your digestive tract. It gets your digestive juices going and enhances your appetite (this is the function of the before-dinner drink called the aperitif!). For people with an irritable bowel, alcohol may cause irritable bowel symptoms such as heartburn, stomach pain, and diarrhea.

We usually advise people to drink alcohol in moderation to minimize the effects of alcohol. Moderate alcohol consumption equals no more than one drink per day for women and no more than two drinks per day for men. One drink is equivalent to 5 ounces (150 ml) of wine, 12 ounces (375 ml) of beer, or 1 1/2 ounces (45 ml) of 80-proof spirits. For the people who cannot drink even a small amount of alcohol without increasing their irritable bowel symptoms, it's best to avoid alcoholic beverages.

We have stated before, it is your choice whether you consume potentially offending foods and beverages, but you need to prepare yourself for the consequences of increased symptoms. Alcohol is unique in that it is a harmful substance if consumed in excess. In addition, some people should not drink alcoholic beverages for specific health reasons such as liver or pancreatic disease, or while taking certain medications. If you do not already know whether it is OK for you to drink alcohol, check with your doctor.

Lactose: The Suspected Sugar?

Another food item that is often the reason for diet adjustments is lactose. Some people cannot tolerate this natural milk sugar. Symptoms of lactose intolerance are gas, bloating, and diarrhea—anywhere from 15 minutes to 2 hours after lactose is consumed.

Milk sugar is normally broken down into smaller sugars and absorbed in the small bowel. People who are lactose intolerant do not break all of the milk sugar down, so that when lactose gets to the large bowel (the last part of your digestive tract), bacteria digest it and produce gasses in the process. This causes people to feel gassy and bloated. Diarrhea occurs because many little sugar molecules (that should not be in the large bowel) attract water to the bowel, and hence watery stools result.

Lactose intolerance is a separate condition from irritable bowel. However, as you can see, it may have similar symptoms—namely, gas, bloating, and diarrhea. In fact, irritable bowel symptoms are frequently mistaken as the result of lactose intolerance. This may lead to the unnecessary avoidance of milk products and potential nutrient deficiencies. We see many people in our clinic who needlessly avoid milk products. It is important to sort out whether you are lactose intolerant or have irritable bowel, or both.

Lactose intolerance can be diagnosed by several tests at your local hospital or health clinic. The two most common are the hydrogen breath test and the lactose tolerance test. Often, it is diagnosed by removing lactose from the diet and assessing whether symptoms go away. This may be a challenge to determine, since lactose intolerance symptoms can be similar to those of an irritable bowel. Still, if you are lactose intolerant, and you remove lactose from your diet, you should feel significantly less gassy and bloated and have less diarrhea.

Generally, people are not 100 percent lactose intolerant. Most people with lactose intolerance can handle small amounts of lactose, such as milk in tea or coffee, the lactose in hard cheese, the milk solids in margarine, and the milk in a piece of cake or muffin. Many people tolerate a small amount of milk (1/2 cup or 120 ml) for cereal and the milk solids present in yogurt.

Determining If You Are Lactose Intolerant If you have the symptoms of gas, bloating, and diarrhea, or loose (watery) stools, you can determine whether you are lactose intolerant by having a test as noted, or you can remove lactose from your diet for a 2- to 3-week trial (see page 47 for information on food tolerance testing).

If you remove lactose-containing foods from your diet, target milk, cream, puddings, yogurt, frozen yogurt, ice cream, and all types of cheese. If you feel you cannot do without milk in your tea or coffee, use low-lactose milk (you can buy this in your local grocery store). Watch to see if your symptoms diminish or go away. If you do not feel any different, lactose intolerance is not the problem; feel free to enjoy a variety of milk products.

If you feel as if you have less bloating, gas, and diarrhea, you may be lactose intolerant. The next step is to determine how lactose intolerant you are. Can you put milk in tea or coffee? Can you have a small amount of milk on your cereal? Can you eat yogurt or enjoy hard cheese? The best way to test this is to try a lactose-containing item in small amounts. It is important that you eat small amounts at a time (see page 47), such as 1 to 2 ounces (30 to 60 g) of hard cheese, 1/2 cup (120 ml) of yogurt, or 1/2 cup (120 ml) of milk with cereal. You may well find that you can enjoy lactose-containing foods in small amounts.

If you are lactose intolerant, it would be wise to choose a low-lactose milk to ensure that you meet your requirement for calcium. Low-lactose milk should be available at your local grocery store. You can also buy a lactase enzyme, which breaks down lactose, at your pharmacy.

Lactose intolerance and milk allergy are not the same thing. People who are allergic to milk have an allergic reaction (a specific chemical response) to the proteins in milk. Milk allergy in adults is very rare. In the case of milk allergy, all milk products need to be avoided, and a calcium supplement is necessary.

Meeting Your Calcium Needs

We find that the majority of female patients who come to our clinic do not consume enough calcium. Actually, this isn't so unusual when you consider that the calcium content of the diet of many North Americans is less than recommended. This is particularly worrisome because a poor calcium intake over time results in weak bones prone to fracture. Compounding this for women is the hormonal change of decreased estrogen at menopause, which causes accelerated loss of calcium from the bone.

A diet deficient in calcium is one of the risk factors for osteoporosis, which is a condition whereby your bones become porous and fragile and may fracture or break easily. One in four women will develop osteoporosis. Increasing calcium just at menopause has a limited effect on preventing osteoporosis, so it's best if you seek calcium early in life, especially for teenagers and adult women.

Milk, cheese, and yogurt are the best sources of calcium. If you do not consume adequate dairy products, it will be difficult to get the calcium your body needs. You may require a calcium supplement. An expert panel of nutrition scientists from Canada and the United States has studied nutrients for bone health and recommends 1,000 milligrams of calcium daily for people between the ages of 19 and 50 and 1,200 milligrams from age 51 to 70; the recommended amount for vitamin D is 200 IU (5 mcg) per day until the age of 50 years and 400 IU (10 mcg) for people between the age of 51 and 70.

Chapter Seven

Stress
How It Affects an
Irritable Bowel

Stress is a familiar word to us all; in fact, so familiar that it has lost any clear meaning. We talk about how we are constantly stressed out and how the world is becoming more and more stressful. But is stress always bad? The answer is NO! So when does manageable stress ("I'm doing OK") or an exciting challenge ("I can't wait to do that again") become overwhelming distress ("I can't take it anymore")?

Although stress is an overused word, we should not overlook the effects it can have on an irritable bowel. In this chapter and the next, we will teach you about stress: how to define it, how to assess your own stress level, and, most importantly, how to reduce stress.

Let's start with some common questions:

1. What does stress mean? Stress is a psychological term that refers to the body's reaction to a challenge or threat. Anything that challenges the body (of which the mind is a part) is stressful. We categorize stress by the primary system that is being challenged. Running up a flight of stairs stresses the muscles and the heart (a physical stress); confronting a critical boss for a raise stresses you psychologically (an emotional stress).

With stress, even though the mind may initially be challenged, the body reacts as well (and vice versa). For example, if you encounter a traffic accident on your way home tonight, you are likely to rush out of your car and lend help, without much thought. Once you get home, though, you might begin to feel distressed. Your initial reaction is physical; after you've had a chance to think about it, the stress becomes psychological.

Psychological stress takes many forms, and it has been repeatedly shown in research studies that stress can affect the functioning of the gut, including the bowel and entire gastrointestinal tract.

2. How does stress affect the gut? When stressed, the body automatically reacts; this is the so-called fight-or-flight response. This reaction is the body's way of getting ready to take action.

Think of your body as a fire department. When a fire alarm sounds, the fire department responds as quickly as possible. All alarms are treated as serious, whether the alarm is false or real.

The body works in much the same way. The stress response is the body's alarm system. When stress is perceived, the body prepares for action—whether there is a need for action (for example, running from a rabid dog who has wandered into the yard) or not (for example, how you feel when your boss unfairly criticizes you but you can do nothing except sit and take it).

In order to prepare you for action, several things happen in your body when under stress. Muscles tighten, your heartbeat and breathing speed up, and stress hormones such as adrenaline are released. Each of these normal reactions can affect your gut. Muscle tension can alter the normal rhythms of your bowel, leading to altered bowel habits (constipation, diarrhea) or to heartburn (see chapter 1).

One way to think about your gut is to imagine a 100-piece orchestra. When all the instruments are working properly and playing in sync (the horns come in when they are supposed to, the drum stops at the right moment), beautiful music results. But if the rhythm is thrown off (the horns play when the drums are supposed to, not all the horns play at the same time), nothing but irritating noise results. This is how the gut works as well. That is why you can have no disease (all the instruments are in good working order) but very intense symptoms that interfere with your ability to function and cope (the orchestra makes nothing but noise).

Because stress has such a strong effect on the body, individuals with an irritable bowel need to be able to manage and reduce stress. This is true both for positive stresses (the challenge of a new job or anxiously awaiting your wedding day) and for negative stresses (losing your job or worrying about finances).

How you manage stress differs according to its type and source. In this book we will talk about three types of stress. First, there is the stress that directly results in irritable bowel symptoms (direct stress effect). Second, there are some people who tend to become worried about their health in general, and irritable bowel is only part of the picture (these individuals are called somatically preoccupied. See chapter 10). Third, there are some people who have psychological problems apart from irritable bowel (these people are identified as having psychopathology. See chapter 10).

Feeling Stressed?

Before we look at each of these types of stress, let's talk about how you can evaluate your own stress level. It is important to accept that stress is subjective. Only you can tell if you are stressed and to what level. This is important because people usually use their own experience to judge others. Problems in relationships ("You just don't understand" or "I don't know why you are upset, it wasn't a big deal") are often due to one person not accepting the other person's experience. Consider bungee jumping. Some people would find this a terrifying experience and think you would have to be out of your mind to do it. Yet others find it exciting and fun. Who is right? No one; it depends on how you experience it.

Take a moment and ask yourself, "How stressed do I feel?" Your answer may depend on whether you are thinking about the past month or the past year. A good time frame to consider is two months. On page 88 you will find "The Stress Test," which will help you recognize your overall stress level, as well as of some of the stress symptoms that bother you. You'll notice that irritable bowel symptoms are not included in this assessment; we assume you have these symptoms because you are reading this book.

The Stress Test

Based on how you have been feeling over the past two months, answer the following questions by circling True or False:

	True	False
Life is exciting	T	F
I wake up feeling refreshed	T	F
I am calm and relaxed	T	F
I feel in control of my life	T	F

Over the past two months, how happy and content have you been? (Circle the number: 1 = Not at all happy; 5 = Extrememly happy)

1   2   3   4   5

Over the past two months, how much have you felt stressed?

1   2   3   4   5

Now, check the following stress symptoms that bother you or interfere with your quality of life. If you experience any symptoms of stress that aren't listed, please note them.

Can't relax	Yes	No
Disturbed sleep	Yes	No
Worry too much	Yes	No
Can't slow down	Yes	No
Always feel I'm behind	Yes	No
Eat to calm myself	Yes	No

Your responses to these questions should reveal your level of stress. But remember, stress is different from person to person.

Exposing the Stressors

Next, using the following chart, list the specific things that you consider the main stresses in your life, especially the things that you find upsetting. Beside each stressor, rate how upsetting the event is, assigning a number from 1 (not at all upsetting) to 10 (extremely upsetting).

For each stressful event, ask yourself whether it is time-limited (for example, an upcoming performance review by your boss) or whether the stress has no foreseeable end (for example, an unemployed federal civil servant looking for another job). Time-limited stressors are acute stressors, and chronic stressors have no clear end. Put an *A* beside the acute stresses and a *C* beside the chronic stresses. Chronic stress is more difficult to manage than acute stress and often has a greater impact on the body because the body can never get away from it (even if you can temporarily shut it out of your mind).

My Stressors

Stress	How Upsetting? (1 to 10) 1=Not Upsetting 10=Very Upsetting	Acute or Chronic? (A or C)
1. _____	_____	_____
2. _____	_____	_____
3. _____	_____	_____
4. _____	_____	_____
5. _____	_____	_____
6. _____	_____	_____

Doing Something About Stress

Can you do anything to alter the stress? It depends on whether it is controllable or not. For example, stress associated with the death of a loved one cannot be altered. On the other hand, if a coworker is insensitive to your needs, you can speak to him or her using assertiveness techniques. (More on this in chapter 8.)

Uncontrollable stressors are more difficult to deal with than controllable ones. If you have many uncontrollable stresses that cause moderate upset or greater, the information starting on page 94 will be especially helpful in learning how to reduce the impact of stress on your body.

If you consider yourself to be stressed, and it has lasted a month or more, ask yourself, "What do I do to cope with stress? And does it work?" In the chart below, list the things you do to cope and then rate if they are successful. For now, do not rate the coping techniques as "positive" or "negative."

My Coping Techniques

What do you do to cope with stress?	Positive (P) or Negative (N)?
1. _____	_____
2. _____	_____

3. _____   _____

4. _____   _____

How well do these strategies work? (1=Not at all; 5=Extrememly well)

                                1   2   3   4   5

What coping strategies would you like to do more of, and what less of?

More Of	Less Of
_____	_____
_____	_____
_____	_____
_____	_____

Note that some coping strategies can be negative and some positive. Positive coping strategies include things like sitting down and analyzing a problem, seeking support from others, and exercising. Negative coping may include things like drinking coffee or alcohol, smoking, and eating to excess. Mark whether your coping strategies are positive (P) or negative (N). It may help to ask friends what they think, because sometimes we deny unhealthy behavior ("I just drink to relax, I can stop anytime").

Is It Daily Hassles or Life?

The final step in assessing your stress level is being aware of the distinction between stress associated with "life events" and stress that comes from daily hassles.

Life event stresses are major events that happen in life that almost anyone would find stressful, things like losing your job, the death of a loved one, getting married, or moving to a new city. These types of stresses usually fall into several categories: finances, relationships, health, and social functioning. These events tend to be relatively easy to identify.

Apart from life's major events, a very common source of stress is daily hassles. These small things that we often ignore can build up and have an accumulated negative effect on our emotions and health. Getting stuck in traffic and being late for an appointment, being treated rudely by a store clerk, and spilling coffee on your new clothes are all small things that can get under our skin.

Since daily hassles are minor, we tend to overlook them. We also do not usually seek social support by talking about them. Too often we're greeted by an unsympathetic ear ("What are you complaining about? Everyone goes though that"). However, these daily hassles can build up and add to our stress.

Self-Monitoring

Most people do not pay close attention to the fine details of their life. For instance, what did you eat for lunch last Wednesday? Unless you eat the same lunch each day, you probably don't remember. There are just too many other things to attend to in a day. Consequently, we don't pay close enough attention and cannot recall small details of our day-to-day activities. Yet learning how to change behavior, and to manage stress, requires being able to identify patterns that are called stress-symptoms associations.

To successfully manage stress, you will need to be able to keep accurate records. We call this self-monitoring. You already have experience with this by completing the symptom, diet, and stress diary in chapter 2. We will help you manage stress by keeping a similar diary, this one much more specific to stress.

Complete the following diary for a two-week interval. Each day, record the intensity of your irritable bowel symptoms, your overall stress level, the stresses of the day, how they affected you in terms of irritable bowel symptoms, feelings, and worries, and how you coped. After two weeks, analyze your stress diary. Look for connections between stress and symptoms, identify the specific stresses that bother you, and identify coping techniques.

We don't recommend that you try to keep a detailed record for more than two weeks because most people find it too difficult to sustain. As well, we don't try to analyze your record until after you've kept it for at least one week. Stress patterns are often subtle and need to be studied over time.

ENLARGE THIS RECORD TO 200% ON YOUR COPIER

Stress Diary

For two weeks, choose a convenient time each day to reflect on the day and identify the extent and source of your stress:

Date	Level of Distress	Stresses of the Day	Irritable Bowel Symptoms	Feelings and Worries	How Did You Cope?

0=none 5=moderate 10=severe

Chapter Eight

Stress Management
Getting the Upper Hand

Stress management is essential to successfully manage an irritable bowel. In this chapter you will learn techniques for coping with stress. For these techniques to be effective, though, be prepared to practice them before you can master them. This is a basic principle to coping skills; practice, practice, practice!

Think of stress reduction skills as you would driving skills. You wouldn't get your beginner's permit on Wednesday, go out for your first driving lesson on Thursday, and expect to pass your driver's exam on Friday. Nor would you go onto the highway in rush hour for your first driving lesson. You would probably start in an empty parking lot. It takes repeated practice to build skill and confidence. It is the same with stress reduction techniques.

When learning stress reduction techniques, you should first practice them when you are calm. Don't expect them to work in stressful situations until you have mastered the technique. Keep in mind that if at first you don't succeed, try, try again.

In this chapter, we discuss the most effective stress management strategies that are available for managing irritable bowel: calming your body, calming your mind, and confronting the stress. We cover a lot of material, so don't worry if you feel that you need to reread sections. In fact, we recommend it. Only by trial and error will you discover how these techniques will work for you, and which is best suited to managing your symptoms.

We provide all the ingredients, and it is up to you to combine them into a stew. Like food, the techniques must fit your taste (not to mention your lifestyle). One thing that is true about stress management techniques: no one technique has been shown to work best for everyone. The best technique is one that makes sense to you, that you can learn to do well, that suits your personality and life situations, and that you can incorporate into your life.

Calming Your Body

As you know, irritable bowel involves a disruption in the normal rhythms of the gut. And stress makes this worse by further disrupting the system. As a result, learning how to calm your body is critical for helping the gut resume its normal, healthy rhythms, thereby reducing your symptoms!

In our experience, it is essential for people with irritable bowel to learn how to keep their bodies calm—especially if their symptoms are the main cause of stress in their lives. Even if you eliminate the cause of your stress, your body might not automatically return to a state of calm. Therefore, you must learn to reduce your body's level of arousal. If successful, you can expect reduced pain, discomfort, and distress, and more normal bowel function (less diarrhea or constipation, bloating, gas, etc.). Two strategies are important to calm your body. First, learning the skill of deep breathing; second, learning muscle relaxation techniques.

Deep Breathing

Stop reading for a moment and take a deep breath.

Now, take another breath.

Pay attention to the parts of your body that move as you breathe. Put your hand on your chest and take another deep breath.... Did your hand move as you breathed in? Take another breath and observe whether your chest moves up as you breathe in....

If your hand or your chest moved up when you breathed in, you are breathing wrong! If you paused, even slightly, between breathing in and out, you are breathing wrong!

In our work, 99 percent of our patients breathe incorrectly at first. Breathing by using your chest muscles does not allow you to take a deep breath. Chest breathing is called shallow breathing. Some people can even hyperventilate by chest breathing, causing a panic attack. We learn to breathe with our chest muscles because it is easy to control these muscles, and shallow breathing makes it easier to talk and breathe at the same time.

There are a number of reasons why deep breathing is so effective for relaxing the body. First, it slows the rate of breathing, which has a very calming effect. Second, deep breathing makes better use of your lung capacity; you get more air in each breath. Because there is more air in the lungs, your heart rate slows down (it doesn't have to move the blood as quickly) and your blood pressure lowers (the blood doesn't have to be forced through your body as hard). So there are both psychological and physical benefits from deep breathing.

To breathe deeply, use your stomach muscles, not your chest muscles. Sit up straight, put both feet on the floor in front of you, put one hand on your chest, as before, and the other hand on your stomach. Now, push in with your lower hand and resist this push.... Feel those muscles? These are the muscles that control deep breathing.

Deep Breathing
Step 1: Breathe **in** through your nose, pushing your stomach **out.**
Step 2: Breathe **out** through your mouth, pulling your stomach **in.**

Notice that your chest muscles are not used in deep breathing. Now take a few minutes, review these instructions, and practice deep breathing. By keeping one hand on your chest and one on your stomach, you can guide yourself through the exercise. Remember:

Keep your chest hand still and allow your stomach hand to move in and out.

You might also want to practice deep breathing by lying flat on your back and placing a small book (a thin paperback is ideal) on your lower stomach (just below your belly button). Make the book go up when you breathe in and down when you breathe out.

Don't be surprised if these deep breathing exercises first make you feel worse, not better. This is because your normal breathing pattern is being disrupted. The solution to this is **practice.** You should not expect this (or any other techniques in this book) to work immediately. Remember, you shouldn't try to learn deep breathing when you are highly stressed. First learn it when you are calm. Once you are skilled at it, then you can use it to reduce stress.

Deep Muscle Relaxation

The second physical technique you need to learn to reduce irritable bowel symptoms is deep muscle relaxation. This technique is very effective for managing pain, especially when combined with imagery (see page 99), because it directly reduces muscle tension. It is also particularly helpful for altered bowel habits.

There are many ways to relax. Some people take long baths, others go for a stroll, others practice tai chi. However, these methods of relaxation are usually difficult to incorporate into a busy day, and we only do them on occasion. As well, many of these techniques produce mental relaxation but not physical relaxation.

Deep muscle relaxation is a brief method of directly relaxing the body by focusing on the muscles themselves. At first, this technique takes 15 to 20 minutes to complete. Once learned, though, you can accomplish relaxation in a much shorter time.

Like deep breathing, you need to become skilled in muscle relaxation before you can expect it to work. In our clinical practice we tell our patients that they should practice relaxation daily for 10 to 14 days when they are calm before they can expect it to work on their irritable bowel symptoms. Two 20-minute practice sessions daily are ideal to promote learning. If you can't fit in two sessions every day, that's OK, but try your best. Giving up too early is a major problem. Think of these coping skills like investing in the bank; you don't get the returns until down the road, but when they come in, they are worth the wait.

Deep muscle relaxation is such an effective technique for managing irritable bowel because it directly affects muscle tension, which disrupts the timing of bowel movement. Muscle tension can also throw off the timing of secretions throughout the stomach and bowel, further contributing to irritable bowel symptoms. Physically relaxing these muscles can allow the normal rhythms of the bowel to resume and in this way reduce symptoms. It has been shown that by inducing a state of "relaxation," the hypersensitivity of the bowel diminishes, thus reducing the intensity of the symptoms.

Learning how to relax involves learning how to detect when your muscles are tense. For example, take your left hand, make a fist, and squeeze slightly, not hard. Pay attention to the sensations associated with this tension. Now, let go of the tension gradually. Now, do this again, only don't squeeze as hard as the first time, and let go of the tension much more slowly.

You can learn to identify tension by learning to scan your body. To start, take a slow deep breath, clear your mind, and focus your attention on your body.

The first time you try this it will be difficult because you will need to divide your attention between the book and following the instruction. After a few times, though, you will get the hang of it and do it without reading. Once you are familiar with these instructions, scan your body with your eyes closed.

Now, your attention is like the beam of a spotlight, and you can control its direction. Focus your attention on the sensations in the bottom of your feet (hold this for 5 seconds).... Now, focus your attention on the sensations in your neck (hold this for 5 seconds).... Now, focus your sensations on your fingers (hold this for 5 seconds).

Notice that as you move your attention from one body part to another, the sensations in that area become stronger and easier to identify. Learning to scan your body in this way will help you identify areas of tension, areas that you can pay special attention to as you learn deep muscle relaxation.

Now, starting at your head, scan your body to identify areas of tension. Focus on your head... now your neck... now your shoulders... your arms... your chest... stomach... back... buttocks... legs... and feet. Do you feel tight, tense, or painful in any of these areas?

Many people report that certain body parts are commonly associated with tension—most often the jaw, top of head, shoulders, and back.

The best way to learn to relax is to learn how to let go of tension in specific muscle groups. To do this, you should first add a small amount of tension to that muscle group. By adding a small amount of tension voluntarily, you can voluntarily let go of that tension. If you add a small amount of tension for a short period (5 to 10 seconds), then let go of that tension very gradually over a longer period (30 to 45 seconds), you will reduce the level of tension in that muscle group below where you started.

Deep Muscle Relaxation—The Basics

To know how to relax, you need to know the following:

1. When muscles are tense. To learn this, practice scanning your body, that is, focusing your attention inward at specific muscle groups.

2. Adding a small amount of tension. It is critical that you do not tense too hard, but just enough to notice an increase.

3. Let go of the tension. This is the payoff. Learning to slowly let go of tension brings immediate relief and calmness. Be sure to let go slowly and smoothly.

Putting It All Together

Find a comfortable place to lie flat (a bed or recliner is perfect), away from noise and distractions. Loosen any tight-fitting clothing and get comfortable. You should read these instructions one or two times to become familiar with them and then try the procedure.

To achieve a relaxed state, you need to work through a series of muscle groups. Each muscle group should be put through the tense/relax cycle twice before moving on.

How to Tense Your Muscles

Muscle Group	Tense by:
Hands/Forearms	Make a fist and squeeze
Shoulders	Lift shoulders
Neck	Push head back into chair or bed
Forehead	Raise eyebrows
Jaw	Clench teeth
Stomach	Tighten stomach
Back	Push back shoulder blades
Buttocks	Tighten buttocks
Thighs/Hamstrings	Tighten upper legs
Feet/Calves	Point toes up or down

Now, tense your hands and forearms (a small amount), study the tension (5 to 10 seconds at the most)... now relax. Slowly let go of the tension, focusing on easing off the tension slowly. Keep in mind the image of a flower, and the petals of a flower opening in the morning sun; they don't open suddenly but gradually and smoothly. This is how you should relax your muscles as well.

Repeat this procedure for each of the muscle groups listed. It should take 20 to 25 minutes to go through them all. It is not important that you feel extremely relaxed afterward, especially the first few times. What is critical is that you can feel some degree of relaxation (that is, you know you are at least more relaxed than when you started). If you can do this, deep relaxation will come with practice.

Imagery

The power of imagination is a form of distraction that can also be used to relax. This makes it especially effective for managing pain as well as reducing the sensation of incomplete emptying that often occurs after going to the bathroom.

Start by going somewhere where you won't be disturbed for 3 to 5 minutes. Read the following instructions several times, until you become familiar with them, and then practice the technique.

Close your eyes and create a picture in your mind's eye. Imagine a calm, relaxing scene, such as lying on a sandy Caribbean beach with the sun warming your skin and the breeze in your hair. In creating this image, use all of your senses. See the white sand and the sun glittering off each tiny grain. See the green-blue of the ocean and hear the wind in the palm trees and the far-off call of seabirds. Smell the salt air. Feel the heat of the sun and the grains of sand under your feet. Taste the salt on your tongue from the sea breeze.

By involving all your senses, you will become more involved in the image, and it will be more distracting to you. Most people find that an image will stay clearly in their mind for 20 to 30 seconds before dissolving. This is normal. When it happens, simply recreate the image by asking yourself the sense questions (what do I hear, see, feel, smell, taste?).

Imagery can be a very useful strategy because your imagination is boundless. Be creative and have fun. The types of images that people most often find useful are relaxing images (like the beach), exciting images (skiing in fresh powder on a sunny day), or detailed images (imagining all the colors in a rainbow).

Use the Relaxation Practice Log on the next page to track the effectiveness of your relaxation sessions. Remember, the more you practice, the more success you will experience.

Exercise: Just Try It

The final physical strategy that will help an irritable bowel is exercise. The body was built to be used, and physical activity is essential for health—both psychological and physical. It helps build healthier bones, and it makes you feel better about yourself. Almost everybody is aware of the many benefits from exercise. So why is it so difficult for many of us to regularly exercise?

Two main barriers seem to get in the way: expectations and lifestyle. We expect too much, either of ourselves (why am I still hurting and breathless?) or of the exercise itself (I should be feeling/looking better by now!). It can also be challenging to fit exercise into a busy lifestyle (see "You Can Do It" below). Yet the benefits of exercise for an irritable bowel are clear.

Physical activity helps calm the body, discharge tension, and reset the body's natural rhythms. Exercise also causes the release of endorphins—a natural substance in the brain that relieves pain and promotes feelings of well-being.

The hardest part about exercising is getting started. This is **the** big hurdle. Once you get started, though, exercise can easily become part of your routine, something you do every day like getting your children off to school, eating lunch with colleagues, or catching the evening news. Even so, exercise, like most activities, needs to be planned and regular. Behavior, when repeated regularly, usually becomes habit in 4 to 6 weeks. Once exercise is a habit it is easier to keep up with it.

You Can Do It!

No time?	Try to rearrange your schedule, then pick a time and stick to it.
Too tired?	Exercise provides energy; it doesn't drain it.
Don't like to exercise?	Make exercise a fun, social event. Set up a reward system to treat yourself. Focus on the health benefits.
Bad weather?	Be flexible, have choices, get wet.

ENLARGE THIS RECORD TO 200% ON YOUR COPIER

Relaxation Practice Log

Date

Skill Used
(Breathing/Muscle Relaxation/Imagery)

How Relaxing?
(0 to 10—"not at all" to "extremely")

| No child care? | Trade off with a friend, use nap time. |
| Too expensive? | Resist treating exercise like a fashion show. |

Exercise gurus say that in order for exercise to be of benefit, you need to be physically engaged in moderate to vigorous activity (see the following chart) at least 30 minutes daily. Where can you find that half hour, and what should you do? Can you find time for a brisk walk in the day? Can you squeeze it in the morning before work, or before your children are awake? Can you walk at lunchtime; convince coworkers to join you? Does your place of work have a worksite exercise program? Can you exercise at the end of a workday, or in the evening? If you cannot exercise daily, can you double your efforts and exercise for an hour to make up for the day you take off. With a bit of creativity and effort, you will be able to overcome the common barriers to exercise.

The best activity to choose is one that you like, and even better, one that will interest a friend or family member to join in. If you live where it's cold part of the year, you may need to find indoor and outdoor activities in order to exercise year-round. In the winter months, try walking in the local shopping mall, enrolling in a low-impact aerobics class, or swimming at a local indoor pool.

Examples of Physical Activity

Moderate*	Vigorous*
brisk walking (3–4 miles/hour)	jogging
gardening	swimming
canoeing	cycling
dancing	racket sports (tennis, squash,
golfing	racquetball)
mowing lawn	hiking
aerobic dance	cycling
using ski or rowing machine	
in-line skating	

*Whether an activity is moderate or vigorous depends largely on the amount of effort expended. For example, cycling can be a moderate activity at less than 10 miles per hour.

It is wise to check with your doctor before you begin any physical activity to ensure the types of activity you choose are safe for you. Also, if you are just starting to exercise or have been away from physical activity for several months or more, a gradual increase in physical activity is recommended. For example, to begin brisk walking, start with a 10 to 20 minute brisk walk daily and increase by 5 minutes per week. Or if you are starting an aerobic dance class, gradually work up to a full effort so that you don't stress your muscles or your heart.

Calming Your Mind

Deep breathing, muscle relaxation, imagery, and exercise can all calm your body and help reduce irritable bowel symptoms. But often it is not enough. It is easy to overlook the great deal of stress that is produced by our tendency to worry or catastrophize (thinking in terms of worst-case scenarios). If you have found the main source of your stress is internal, focus on calming your mind.

A large number of clinical studies have demonstrated that thinking patterns strongly influence emotions, behavior, and bowel symptoms. By monitoring your stress reactions and looking for thoughts associated with symptoms, or with feelings of stress, you can identify patterns of thinking that contribute to irritable bowel symptoms. Knowing this, you can work to alter your thinking style.

This is not simply the power of positive thinking. It is a method of analyzing our thoughts and thinking them through from a different perspective. Three steps are involved: self-monitoring, self-analysis, and cognitive restructuring.

Self-Monitoring

Like so many other aspects of managing an irritable bowel, you need to study your own situation to learn how your symptoms are produced and, ultimately, controlled. By keeping a record of irritable bowel episodes and stressful events, with an eye toward identifying thinking patterns, you can determine how much work you need to do on your thinking patterns.

To do this you need to attend to the content of your thoughts (stream of consciousness). It takes some time and effort to analyze thought patterns. In fact, it is best to write them down (see page 105). That's because thought patterns become routine, and as they do, they become difficult to recognize. They can also disguise true feelings; thoughts become shorthand in nature. For example, each time a friend asks you out for dinner, you think, "Oh no, I can't," which is shorthand for, "Oh no, I can't. If I go I may have uncontrollable gas and humiliate myself." Notice the translation required to go from the experienced thought to the underlying meaning.

When you note your thoughts, it helps to put them in the form of statements, not questions. ("What if I have gas?" usually means, "I will have gas and humiliate myself.") It is also useful to keep in mind that thoughts can occur as words (self-talk) or images (picturing yourself making smelly gas at a busy restaurant and people turning to look).

Finally, to help you learn to identify stress-related automatic thoughts, ask yourself the following question when you are recording your thoughts: What was upsetting me in this situation? Don't apply logic and reason when answering this question. Base your answer on your distressing feelings.

For the following form, we recommend that you use the A-B-C method. A refers to the activating event (the situation that brought on your stress/symptoms), and C refers to the emotional and behavioral consequences. Between A and C is B, your beliefs or thoughts in the situation.

Think back over the past week or two and identify a situation in which you either felt stress or had an episode of irritable bowel symptoms that you believe was stress related. Take a moment and recall the details of the situation. The more you note, the better. Now write down the situation in the first column of the chart on page 105. In the third column, write down your feelings. In the second column, write down the thoughts that were associated with your distress. After you have recorded your thoughts and feelings for four or five days, you will be ready to analyze your thought patterns and change any harmful ones.

Self-Analysis

After you have kept the record for four or five days, sit down and analyze the results. Do you see a tendency toward negative thinking? Are you worrying about how things will work out, or your ability to cope? If so, you will need to learn to confront and challenge negative thinking styles.

ENLARGE THIS RECORD TO 200% ON YOUR COPIER

Thoughts Into Action

A Situation
(when, what, who, where?)

B Automatic Thoughts
(what you were thinking at the time)

C Feelings
(how did it make you feel?)

Cognitive Restructuring

Certain thinking styles are associated with distress. And learning about these styles can help you alter your thoughts. Psychologists call this cognitive restructuring, a technical term that refers to the process of changing, or restructuring, thoughts. It often involves learning how to realistically evaluate situations in a way that helps rather than harms.

It's easy to become overwhelmed and feel like giving up when facing the unpleasant symptoms of an irritable bowel. Unfortunately, not only do negative thoughts affect your mental state, but they can affect your physical state, causing symptoms to worsen. This makes restructuring your thoughts and maintaining a realistic optimism all the more important. Cognitive restructuring is helpful for a number of irritable bowel symptoms: altered bowel habits, the worry that often accompanies mucus in the stool and abdominal bloating, and the sensation of incomplete emptying after going to the bathroom.

Once you have identified your negative, stress-inducing thoughts, confront them! Challenge your negative thinking. Ask yourself:

- Are there any other ways of thinking about this?
- If I was giving advice to a friend who was thinking this, what would I say?
- If I can't change the situation, how can I live with it?

Cognitive restructuring can be challenging to learn, and most people give up easily. It seems that negative thinking styles, once they set in, are automatic and more easily embraced than coping thoughts, especially at first. With practice, however, coping thoughts become more believable. This is particularly true if you can prove your old way of thinking is wrong.

Turning Negatives Into Positives

Negative Thinking Style	Definition
Catastrophizing	Thinking in terms of worst-case scenarios. Often expressed as "what if" thoughts.
Black and White Thinking	Thinking that situations are either all good or all bad with little in between.
Magnifying/Minimizing	Overemphasizing negative events and underemphasizing positive ones.

| Selective Attention | Focusing only on the negative or stressful aspects of a situation, ignoring the rest. |
| Personalizing | Thinking that bad things reflect your character rather than just luck or circumstances. |

Reducing the Stress

Up to this point we have talked about what you can do to reduce the impact of stress by calming your body and calming your mind. Equally important, however, is to reduce the stress whenever possible. This is especially important if the majority of your stress stems from external forces such as your job, family, or friends.

As mentioned earlier, there are two types of stressful situations: controllable and uncontrollable. Uncontrollable stress results from events that you, or no one else, can do anything about. The death of a loved one, losing your job, or having your house burn down are uncontrollable stresses. Here you need to accept the stress and minimize its impact on you.

Controllable stresses might be things like being unemployed (you might not be able to control losing your job, but you can try to get another), conflict in a relationship, or being overwhelmed at work. By controllable, we don't mean that you have total control; we do mean that there are things you can do to influence the outcome. You need to take action to help manage controllable stress.

Learning the difference between controllable and uncontrollable stresses is very difficult. Ask yourself, "Is there anything I might be able to do about this situation?" Or, "Does everyone react to this stress the same way, or do other people do something different?" It is also helpful to ask a trusted person if he or she considers your stress issue controllable or not. Often, others can see some action we could take that we are unable to see.

We recommend using the following strategies when trying to change the stress in your life:

- Problem solving (brainstorm, evaluate pros/cons, pick solution, try it out, evaluate)
- Time management (set realistic priorities and limits, plan for relaxation)
- Assertiveness (broken record, fogging)

Problem Solving

If you are going to try to work through a problem, pick a time when you are relatively calm, have some time, and aren't preoccupied with other things. Going to a different setting often helps, for instance, the park on a sunny day, a favorite coffee shop, or some other situation that takes you out of your routine. We can often think more clearly about a situation when we are removed from it. Be sure to have a pen and paper.

Step 1: Write down the problem in a clear, brief manner.

Step 2: Write down what you'd like to see happen; what is your realistic goal?

Step 3: Brainstorm. Write down all possible solutions, without evaluating any. Don't worry how silly or unfeasible the solution seems; just get it down on paper.

Step 4: Now, go back and consider each possible solution. Give each careful thought before dismissing it. Be sure to blend and modify as you go through the list.

Step 5: Pick the best solution from the list.

Step 6: Write down the advantages and disadvantages of following through on this solution. You might want to discuss this option with a trusted other to get someone else's opinion.

Step 7: Follow through on this solution.

Step 8: Evaluate the outcome of your solution. How did it work?

Step 9: Return to step 1 if you are not satisfied with the results.

Time Management

A great deal of stress that contributes to irritable bowel is produced by living a hectic lifestyle in which we try to cram as much as we can into the limited time we have. As a result, managing our time is extremely important. This involves three main issues: setting realistic goals, prioritizing (which really means deciding that we will not get some things done), and building relaxation into our plan.

Sit down with pen and paper. Make a list of the tasks you will face next week. Now, consider how much time each will reasonably take and how much time you have. (It may be a good idea to multiply your time estimate by 1.5, as most tasks take longer than we plan). Now make sure you plan in time to eat your meals leisurely, and to use relaxation methods. Remember: Plan your work and work your plan!

Assertiveness

Our experience in working with stress issues in general, and stress-related bowel symptoms in particular, is that relationships are a major source of stress. Therefore, we want to give you two very useful techniques for dealing with difficult people. These are verbal techniques that will help you get your point across without getting angry, or pulled into an argument, and also help you deal with negative comments by others. These techniques are called the broken record and fogging.

The Broken Record. This technique will help if you want to make a point but don't believe that the person you are talking to wants to hear. In such situations, most people try to explain and justify themselves. For instance, if you say, "I don't think I'll be able to work late tonight," and your boss responds, "But I'll only need you for an hour, maybe less, so I'm sure you can swing that," you might be tempted to explain yourself ("But I told my husband I'd get dinner started early tonight"). This is not a great response because it leaves you open for a counterresponse ("Why don't you just get takeout, I know you like Burger King"). You then need to come back with another explanation. And if the other person doesn't really want to hear you, you will usually run out of explanations before they run out of pressuring comments.

To avoid this, use the broken record technique. Like a broken record, repeat the same thing (word for word) over and over again, regardless of what the other person says. If you can prepare, think of what you want to say in the most direct way, using as few words as possible and a polite tone. Then just repeat this over and over. After three or four repetitions, the other person gets the message.

Try this with a friend. Set up a role-play in which your friend asks you to deliver a parcel. You respond with, "Sorry, but I won't be able to do it." Ask your friend to give you a hard time about this. Once you've tried this once or twice, you'll see how liberating it is.

Fogging. The broken record technique, and communication in general, would be much easier if the person you were talking to kept silent and listened. Inevitably, however, the other person has something to say, and it's often what you don't want to hear. You can't just ignore what the other person says, and very often your response escalates the conflict. Consider the following exchange:

> Person A: I have to leave early, and the boss needs this in a half hour, so I'll leave it on your desk. Thanks.
>
> Person B: Sorry, but I've got a deadline as well from Debbie, so I won't be able to do it.
>
> Person A: But I'm sure yours can wait. This is really important, and I can't miss my appointment. I know Debbie is out this afternoon, so if you get it to her first thing tomorrow, I'm sure it will be fine.
>
> Person B: I've got a deadline as well, so I won't be able to do it. Debbie gave me two things to do, so I won't have time tomorrow.
>
> Person A: But you can stay late. You said the kids are staying with your parents.
>
> Person B: Yeah, but I wanted to do some shopping on the way home.
>
> Person A: I heard there is a big sale at the mall starting tomorrow, so why don't you go then?
>
> Person B: I can't go tomorrow. Brian has a game.
>
> Person A: But the games don't start until 6. Why are you being so difficult? How can shopping be more important than this appointment? You know I haven't been feeling well; I thought you were my friend.
>
> Person B: I am. Just leave the memo and I'll try to get to it.
>
> Person A: Thanks, you're great!
>
> Person B: No problem. (Inside she's thinking, No I'm not; I'm a sucker.)

Does this scenario sound familiar? The situation is typical in that Person A is trying to control Person B in order to solve her own problem. Person B did OK for the first two comments (she stuck with the broken record), but things went haywire when she started to respond to the specifics of what Person A said. As the conversation continued, Person B's point (I have my own deadline) got forgotten. Person A simply got more pushy, finally questioning the friendship. At that point, Person A caved in and agreed to do the work.

How could you avoid falling into this trap? By using the fogging technique. Fogging is the art of agreeing without actually agreeing. Sound confusing? It really isn't. To avoid escalating conflict in a situation like this, find something in what the person said and acknowledge or agree with it—without agreeing to the behavior the person wants from you (for example, "I can understand that's how you feel." Or, "You may be right."). Also, be sure to use the broken record technique each time you respond. Let's go through the scenario again, this time using the fogging technique.

> Person A: I have to leave early, and the boss needs this in a half hour, so I'll leave it on your desk. Thanks.
>
> Person B: Sorry, but I've got a deadline as well from Debbie, so I won't be able to do it.
>
> Person A: But I'm sure yours can wait. This is really important, and I can't miss my appointment. I know Debbie is out this afternoon, so if you get it to her first thing tomorrow, I'm sure it will be fine.
>
> Person B: I understand that it's important, and you can't miss your appointment, but I've got a deadline as well, so I won't be able to do it.
>
> Person A: But you can stay late. You said the kids are staying with your parents.
>
> Person B: Yeah, that's true, but I've got a deadline as well, so I won't be able to do it.
>
> Person A: But your deadline can't be more important than mine.
>
> Person B: That may be true, but I've got a deadline as well, so I won't be able to do it.
>
> Person A: Why are you being so difficult? You know I haven't been feeling well. I thought you were my friend.
>
> Person B: I can see why you think I'm being difficult, but I've got a deadline as well, so I can't do it.

Person A: Are you sure there is no way you can do it?

Person B: Sorry, but I've got a deadline as well, so I won't be able to do it.

Person A: OK, I'll see if Bob can do it.

Notice the difference between the two scenarios. In the second, Person B did not lose sight of her point; she consistently used the broken record. By doing so, she did not get dragged into a debate about other points. And by using fogging, she was able to respond politely and acknowledge Person A. Person B needed to use the broken record and fogging four or five times consecutively until Person A backed down (which is realistic, in our experience), but Person B did not give in.

These verbal techniques (broken record and fogging) take practice before they can be used comfortably. The practice is well worth it, however, as these techniques can eliminate a lot of stress brought on by people making unreasonable demands on you.

Practice Log for Broken Record/Fogging Techniques

Use this form to keep track of your experiences learning to use the broken record and fogging techniques. In choosing situations to try these techniques, identify an actual event or stage an artificial situation in which you ask someone to role-play with you.

Hint: At first it might help to write down what you would like to say for the broken record and keep this handy. Remember, say the same thing over and over. Also, create a list of fogging statements that you could use in a variety of situations. Several "stock" statements can be used in most situations. Examples of fogging statements include:

I can see why you would say that • You might be right • I can see that you want me to _____ • I can see your point

Situation	Broken Record Statement	Fogging Statements	How Well Did It Work? (0–10)

Chapter Nine

What Do I Do About the Pain?

Pain is the most common symptom of an irritable bowel, and the symptom most likely to cause a person to seek medical attention. This is because we all interpret pain as a sign that something is seriously wrong with our body. As well, most of us believe that the intensity of pain reflects the seriousness of harm. However, while your pain can be very severe and is very real (not just "in your head"), it is not causing any damage to your bowel (it hurts but does not harm).

Making the distinction between hurt and harm is very important in pain management. You can learn to live with hurt. The pain will make you feel bad, but it does not mean that any damage is being done to the bowel or that your symptoms will lead to a serious bowel disease (such as colitis or bowel cancer). But how do you learn to live with pain?

In learning to manage pain, you first need to train yourself to recategorize your pain; that is, change how you view the pain and the things that you say to yourself while you are in pain. The automatic reaction to pain is to become alarmed. After all, pain is literally one of the body's alarm systems. If you become familiar enough with your pain (so that you know the difference between regular hurt and unexplained symptoms that might indicate harm), and are adequately reassured that the pain is not harmful, you can learn to remain calm and work with your pain, not against it. Critical to doing this is distinguishing hurt from harm.

Hurt versus Harm

Hurt refers to the experience of pain that is not damaging. For instance, take the muscle pain experienced after a strenuous workout. This is clearly pain, but it does not cause any damage.

By *harm* we refer to pain that is an indication of damage being done. If you've just undergone surgery, pain around the incision when you move is often a sign to stop so that you avoid damage; for example, tear the stitches or staples open. The pain of an irritable bowel hurts but does not harm. It is OK to experience this pain. In fact, by making it OK (a decision you make), you will find that you can work with your pain, not against it.

Our experience in treating people with chronic pain is such that upon successful treatment, the individual says, "You know, I still have the pain, but it is not as bad as before, and it doesn't upset me as it used to. Now I manage the pain, rather than it managing me."

How do you decide what pain is hurtful and not harmful? This first requires a proper diagnosis of your condition as irritable bowel (see chapters 1 and 2). Then you need to ask yourself, "Is this pain familiar? Is it the typical pain I experience with my irritable bowel?" If it is, then recognize the pain as hurt, not harm (even if the pain is intense and continues to alarm you). If your pain is new or changes dramatically, then you may need to consult your doctor to help evaluate whether the pain reflects hurt or harm.

Initially, you should see your doctor about whether your pain is due to the irritable bowel or some other problem or disease. There are nine things that your doctor will want to know about the pain. These features will also help you to better identify things you may be doing that will make the pain better or worse.

Pain Features to Note

1. Where is the pain?
2. Does the pain go anywhere else, such as the back, shoulder, etc.?
3. What does the pain feel like? Common descriptions of pain are sharp like a knife, burning, gnawing, cramping, etc.
4. How long does the pain last?

5. Have you noticed anything that reduces the pain? For instance, lying down, drinking milk or taking an antacid, rubbing your abdomen, or using an ice pack or hot pack?
6. Have you noticed anything that worsens the pain or triggers it? For instance, eating, bending over or lifting heavy objects, bowel motions, etc.?
7. What have you been doing when the pain started?
8. Has the pain ever wakened you from a deep sleep?
9. Have you ever had pain of a similar quality or pattern in the past, even if it was some years ago?

How to Manage the Pain

Pain is a very personal experience. Under different circumstances you will experience different pain levels to the same stimulation. We have all heard of situations where someone has hurt themselves but experienced little pain. The athlete who injures himself or herself during a game often keeps playing without feeling pain. But when the game ends, the pain starts. If that same injury occurred in a car accident, or when falling down the stairs, you can bet that the pain would be worse. The actual damage may not be worse, but the experience of pain would be worse.

Pain intensity (as perceived) is influenced by attention and distress. The more you focus on the pain, the more it upsets you and the more intense it feels. It works the other way, too. The more the pain upsets you, the more you focus on it. Only you experience the intensity of your pain, and therefore it is important to understand the factors that will influence how intensely you will experience your pain. Understanding this will help you better manage your pain.

Pain can vary in its intensity depending on your state of mind. If you are a person that spends your time monitoring your body for symptoms (see chapter 10), then you will tend to experience pain more intensely than other people. It is similar to the football player who breaks a bone in his foot during the fourth quarter of a crucial game. Because he is so focused on winning, he barely notices the pain. Yet he needs crutches to be able to leave the locker room after the game. If that same individual had the same injury while doing something less intense, he would immediately find the pain intolerable. This is important to understand about pain. The injury in both instances is the same, yet the experience of the pain is quite different. By learning techniques that help you to be distracted from—or less aware of—the pain, you will be able to manage your pain better without always resorting to pain medications.

Pain Medications

Many people with irritable bowel try medications to relieve pain. Medications for pain are of two types: narcotic painkillers that are very effective for acute pain, and medications that appear to modify the pain over the longer term, which are more effective for chronic pain.

Narcotic painkillers should never be used for the abdominal pain of irritable bowel. These drugs are addictive and negatively affect the gut. Narcotic painkillers tend to cause constipation and increased abdominal contractions or spasms that actually worsen the pain. What's more, this side effect persists longer than the painkilling effect of the medication. This leads to a vicious cycle for the patient, who seeks increasing doses of the painkiller in the mistaken belief that after receiving "enough" medication, the pain will go away. Unfortunately, what usually happens is that the pain is only temporarily eased. It then returns, often with increased intensity due to the increased bowel contractions and spasms that these drugs accentuate. Some individuals can never receive enough medication to relieve the pain; that is, they are "addicted" to pain medication.

Fortunately, there is a better approach to managing pain with medications, especially if you continue to have frequent and recurrent pain despite practicing techniques to ease the intensity of the pain.

Antidepressants are a group of drugs with a beneficial side effect for many people with an irritable bowel. They ease chronic pain. Although not everyone will see improvement, these medications can be very beneficial for persistent pain.

When antidepressant drugs are used for chronic pain, they are usually prescribed at much lower doses than are used for treating depression. Your doctor has to prescribe these drugs, so you will have to discuss with her the best drug for you. Other medical problems may make antidepressants inappropriate or potentially dangerous.

If your doctor agrees that an antidepressant drug may be helpful for you, consider these points:

- Antidepressants work best for chronic pain.
- Unlike typical painkillers that relieve pain almost immediately, antidepressants are taken daily, usually at night with the dose gradually increased every four to seven days until the pain eases.

Like all medication, antidepressants do have side effects, and you must see your doctor regularly for monitoring while taking them. Still, many people with irritable bowel tolerate antidepressants well. Because the dosage is often much lower than the dose needed to treat depression, they can be taken for prolonged periods to achieve good pain control.

Another group of medications used for pain with irritable bowel are anti-spasm drugs that decrease the contractions and spasms of the bowel. These drugs have limited usefulness for many people with irritable bowel, but some individuals find them helpful for episodes of bowel spasm. Again, these drugs have to be obtained by prescription, so you will have to see your doctor about whether or not one of these drugs may be helpful for the pain. Because these drugs decrease the contractions of the bowel to reduce pain, they can have other side effects such as worsening constipation symptoms.

If you find medication helpful, you should also try pain management techniques like those on the next page and in chapter 8. Don't rely on medication alone to resolve your pain completely.

Other Sources of Pain

Some types of pain cannot be effectively treated with medications or coping techniques. For instance, if you review your symptom diary from chapter 2 and find that there rarely seems to be any aggravating or relieving factors to your pain, it is likely you do not have an irritable bowel but rather a condition called "chronic functional abdominal pain." This condition usually requires expert advice and intensive therapy that is beyond the scope of this book. Still, you may find that some of the techniques in chapters 8 and 10 will help you manage your pain better.

Finally, there are people who suffer with an irritable bowel who have a past history of sexual and/or physical abuse. Such people often have severe pain as part of their symptoms. If this is your situation, it is important to acknowledge that sexual abuse has happened and to seek professional help for the abuse. It is unlikely that you will be able to properly manage your pain and other bowel symptoms until you have addressed the unresolved psychological pain and injury that results from this abuse. We encourage you to speak to your doctor or seek help from a psychologist or psychiatrist or other mental health therapist experienced in dealing with abuse.

Pain Management Strategies

There are three steps to controlling pain: controlling your thoughts, controlling your body, and controlling your behavior.

Controlling Your Thoughts

This strategy is similar to the general coping strategies covered in chapter 8. You need to be able to talk yourself through pain episodes. We need to emphasize again that the normal response of the body to pain is to go into alarm mode. Pain produces an automatic reaction, just like a reflex. This involves focusing your attention on the pain and preparing your body for action, which primarily involves increased muscle tension. When an immediate action cannot be taken to alleviate the pain, you become distressed. This increases your body tension and focuses you even more clearly on your pain. This is what we call the pain cycle. Your job is to prevent your body from automatically going into alarm mode when your irritable bowel pain begins.

To Control Your Thoughts

1. Understand what is happening. You will need to repeat to yourself, over and over until you believe that the pain is not a sign of something terribly wrong but just a sign that you have an irritable bowel (it hurts, but it doesn't harm).

2. Accept chronic pain. You will need to make friends with your pain. Yes, you heard us right, make friends with your pain! Since the pain is produced by your normal bowel, then the pain is normal for you. This is why you may need to consider some pain medication and also why you need to stop the pain cycle.

3. Talk yourself through the pain. When you are in pain, you will automatically become upset and focused on the pain. You will need to work hard to talk yourself through this. Most people find that they benefit from self-statements that keep things in perspective. Telling yourself things like:

- The pain scares me, but I know there is nothing really wrong.
- Don't worry about the pain, just relax and focus on something else.
- I've had this same pain many times before, and it always goes away after a while.
- The more I focus on the pain, the worse it is.

Controlling Your Body

Pain is an alarm signal, and the body, like the fire department, responds to all alarms, even false alarms. The body's response to alarm is to increase muscle tension, heart rate, and blood pressure and to secrete stress hormones. If you want to reduce your pain you will need to learn to control this bodily response. The best way to do this is with relaxation techniques.

Review and practice the relaxation techniques presented in chapter 8. Remember that it is very difficult to use relaxation techniques when in pain (it's like trying to stay calm when the house is on fire), so master them when you are calm, before episodes of pain. You will need to be patient and not give up on relaxation.

Controlling Your Behavior

Because your pain hurts but does not harm, it helps to do things other than focusing on the pain. Distracting yourself is very useful. Do some housework, gardening, or other physical activity that occupies your mind. If there's an opportunity to read, do so; or you might find it helpful to talk with someone. Doing something productive is also helpful in controlling behavior. Not only is it distracting, but the sense of accomplishment when you finish is uplifting as well.

Pain can also be influenced by minimizing some behaviors. First, avoid isolating yourself. Isolation not only encourages you to focus on your pain; it is depressing, which increases suffering. Second, avoid overrelying on medication. As we discussed earlier, medication can be a useful part of your treatment, but do not expect it to cure you. Even if you find medication helpful, you will still need to find other ways of managing your pain.

Chapter Ten

When an Irritable Bowel Is Not Your Only Worry

No one has to tell you that an irritable bowel is a significant management problem in its own right. Unfortunately, some of our patients suffer from additional problems. There are two psychological problems commonly seen with irritable bowel that we will cover in this chapter: worry, anxiety, and preoccupation with your health; and emotional distress, such as clinical depression.

Are You Preoccupied With Your Health?

Most of us don't give much thought to our health—until we face a medical problem. Some people, however, are preoccupied with their health despite having no diagnosed health problems or even health risks. They are prone to worry about any and every body sensation.

If you are overly focused on your body and overly concerned about being ill, you are somatically preoccupied.

We all are aware of our bodies, but mostly we focus on our bodies only when we experience a sensation that is unexpected and uncomfortable. People with somatic preoccupation spend too much time focused on their body. As a result, they are aware of sensations that have no real significance and would not be perceived by others. This is a problem because if anyone focuses their attention internally on their body, the strength of body sensations increases. Worrisome sensations grow in intensity.

To demonstrate this phenomenon, take a moment to focus on the sensations in your feet, where they are resting on the ground (take 15 to 20 seconds to do this now).... Now focus on the sensations in your fingers.... Now the sensations in your neck. Notice that as you move your attention from one part of the body to another, the sensations in that body part become stronger.

Now, focus your attention inward to your body. Starting at the top of your head, scan down to the tips of your toes. Imagine that your attention is like a spotlight that shines on your body. Spend a minute doing this and identify the part of your body that is in the most discomfort. Surprisingly, you will almost always be able to identify an uncomfortable sensation somewhere. Now focus on this sensation. Clear your mind of other thoughts and zero in on this discomfort. As you do this, notice that the sensation gets stronger.

If you are not somatically preoccupied, you will notice a slight increase in the strength of this sensation, but it will quickly fade as your attention turns to other things. If you have a tendency to be somatically preoccupied, you will have more trouble switching your attention away from this sensation. You may even experience a slight increase in feelings of anxiety. However, because you have identified this sensation by following these instructions, this sensation is likely to be mild and easily dismissed. If you became aware of this sensation spontaneously while you were going about your day, the discomfort would be more intense and harder to dismiss.

This attention to bodily sensations is called body vigilance. If you are somatically preoccupied, you are highly vigilant to your body. You notice body sensations more easily than others and perceive these sensations as more intense than others would.

Body vigilance is one key psychological ingredient in somatic preoccupation. The other is the tendency to catastrophize. As we explained in chapter 7, catastrophizing is the tendency to think in worst-case scenarios, in this case, concerning your health. If you are somatically preoccupied, you might think that you are developing a serious disease (cancer) when you perceive a body discomfort.

Not only does somatic preoccupation cause unnecessary upset, it can cause problems in relationships. Others may dismiss your complaints or belittle you. Even doctors aren't immune to poorly treating those who are somatically preoccupied. So how can you reduce the distress brought on by somatic preoccupation? We recommend three things:

1. Reduce Body Stress. Chronic muscle tension directly increases distress because it produces stronger body sensations that can be focused upon and interpreted catastrophically. For instance, take your left hand, make a fist, and squeeze very tightly. Hold your hand in this position until you start to feel a dull ache; it shouldn't take too long. This pain is very real and hard to ignore, yet it is insignificant. It conveys no risk to your health. Yet, as explained in chapter 9, pain is the body's alarm system and very difficult to ignore.

Learning to relax can be very effective in reducing the tendency to overfocus on the body by reducing physical sensations. See page 96 for relaxation exercises.

2. Cognitive Restructuring. It will also help to try to convince yourself that the sensations you feel are not significant. Of course, this is much easier said than done. The cognitive restructuring techniques presented on page 106 will help. You may also find it beneficial to establish a series of self-statements that will help you reduce both hyper-vigilance and catastrophization. We recommend regular practice using the following self-statements or any others that you find effective:

- I know I tend to worry about my health, but I need to get over it.
- Don't worry about this feeling, just relax and focus on something else.
- I've had this same worry many times before, and it always turns out to be nothing.
- The less I worry about it, the less it will bother me.

3. Medical Management. If you are somatically preoccupied, you likely have a strong need for reassurance that nothing is wrong. The best and often the only place to get this reassurance is from your physician. Unfortunately, repeated trips to the doctor about fears that are dismissed can quickly become frustrating for both you and your doctor. Your doctor may even use medical investigations to reassure you. Often this backfires; it increases, not decreases, your concern. Your doctor might say, "I don't think there is anything to worry about, but just to be sure I'll send you for an X ray" (with the expectation that a normal X ray will settle you). However, you might think, "I knew something was wrong. He's just saying I shouldn't worry to ease the blow. He wouldn't order an X ray if he didn't think there was something seriously wrong."

Even if you do receive reassurance as to your health, it can wear off quickly. You might feel good leaving your doctor's office, but by the next day, your concerns are back. We see people who are almost addicted to reassurance. Also, you might fall into the trap of seeking additional medical opinions. The unfortunate fact of medicine, which involves a significant amount of judgment, is that if you consult with five doctors about the same problem, you will hear different opinions. This could reflect different ways of saying the same thing or different interpretations. Nonetheless, it reinforces anxiety and somatic preoccupation.

To avoid this we recommend that you find a physician that you can trust; one you believe takes you seriously and is concerned about you. You and your physician should establish a set schedule of medical appointments, perhaps one every four weeks. Between appointments, you should try coping on your own, using the foregoing strategies. At each appointment, voice your concerns and ask your physician to provide medical feedback. Consulting other doctors should be minimized, as should investigations. Only if your doctor, not you, believes a consultation or investigation is necessary should it take place (this is why you need to trust your doctor).

This strategy can be very effective, since you know that you will see your doctor soon and he or she will listen to you and take you seriously. It also works for your doctor because he or she will know what to expect and not feel that you are overusing the medical system just for reassurance.

Psychopathology:* Overwhelming Emotional Distress

While some people experience irritable bowel in the context of a general tendency to worry about their health (somatic preoccupation), others experience irritable bowel in the context of significant emotional distress (such as clinical depression). This type of emotional distress is referred to as psychopathology.

Fortunately, few people with irritable bowel have such emotional disorders. The purpose of this section is to outline the most common emotional disorders seen with irritable bowel: depression, anxiety disorder, and substance abuse disorder. (For information on chronic abdominal pain associated with past sexual abuse, see page 120.) If you suspect that you have any of the following emotional disorders, we strongly recommend that you seek help from a licensed mental health practitioner, preferably a psychiatrist or a psychologist. Your family doctor may be able to recommend someone to you.

Depression

Everyone gets sad from time to time, and having a chronic condition like irritable bowel can certainly wear away at your optimism and cheer. Sometimes, however, the sadness dominates and becomes a serious problem in itself. This is what we refer to as clinical depression.

It can be difficult to distinguish normal periods of sadness (the blues) from clinical depression, especially in people who have medical symptoms, or for whom depressing events have recently occurred (losing a job, divorce, etc.). It is often helpful to get feedback from a loved one, your family doctor, or a psychologist or psychiatrist if you think your sadness might be problematic. Clinical depression is likely if your sadness is intense, long lasting, and interferes with your ability to function.

Here are some of the signs to look for if you are concerned that you may be depressed. Place a check mark in each box that applies to you. If you check two or more boxes you might want to seek professional help or talk to your doctor about seeking help.

---

*Conditions of psychopathology are specified in the *American Psychiatric Association's Diagnostic and Statistical Manual of Mental Disorders: Fourth Edition* (DSM-IV;1994). The conditions described in this section are consistent with the diagnostic labeling and criteria specified in the DSM-IV.

Sad Mood

In the past 2 weeks or more, have you been feeling sad, down, and
blue most of the time? . . . . ._____

Has this sadness been present for most of the past 6 months? . . . . ._____

Does your mood stay down even if something pleasant happens? . . . . . ._____

Sleep Problems (associated with your sad mood)

Has your sleep been abnormal (trouble falling or staying asleep,
waking early and not being able to get back to sleep, not feeling
rested after sleep)? . . . . ._____

Most nights, are you sleeping 2 or more hours less than normal
for you? . . . . ._____

Most nights, are you sleeping more than normal for you? . . . . ._____

Appetite Problems (associated with your sad mood)

Are you eating more than normal? . . . . ._____

Are you eating less than normal? . . . . ._____

Have you lost weight as a result of your appetite (provided you are
not on a weight loss diet)? . . . . ._____

Energy Problems (associated with your sad mood)

Do you feel tired all the time? · . . . . ._____

Have you lost your interest in things? . . . . ._____

Have you lost motivation to do things? . . . . ._____

Thinking Problems (associated with your sad mood)

Is your ability to concentrate worse than normal? . . . . ._____

Do you feel that your memory is poorer than normal? . . . . ._____

Hopelessness (associated with your sad mood)

Have you been having thoughts and feelings that life is not
worth living? . . . . ._____

Have you thought about ending your life? . . . . ._____

Have you recently had thoughts of taking your life? . . . . ._____

Do you have a plan for taking your life? . . . . ._____

Have you made preparations for taking your life? . . . . ._____

Have you begun to say your good-byes? . . . . ._____

Do you intend to take your life soon? . . . . ._____

Talk to your family doctor or seek professional help if you
have any of the warning signs of depression, particularly if you
are thinking about ending your life.

If you think you or a loved one is clinically depressed, what
can you expect? Although many people are reluctant to see a
mental health professional, you should realize that depressions
are common, treatable conditions that can happen to anybody. It

does not mean that you are weak. There are a number of psychological and medical treatments that are highly effective for treating depressions. Your doctor can help you decide on the best course of treatment for you and can often recommend a good psychiatrist or psychologist. Antidepressant medications are highly effective for treating most depressions, and psychotherapy (such as cognitive behavioral or interpersonal therapy) is also an effective treatment option. Above all, don't suffer silently.

Anxiety Disorders

As with sadness, we all get anxious and worried at times. Indeed, anxiety is a very common factor underlying irritable bowel, as you have learned in this book. Still, some people are so dominated by anxiety that it is a major interference in their life. There are several subtypes of anxiety disorders that you should be aware of: panic, generalized anxiety, obsessive-compulsive syndrome, and post-traumatic stress.

Panic refers to the sudden, intense onrush of anxiety that can't be ignored. It's like going from 0 to 60 in 2.1 seconds. People who have had a panic attack usually remember it vividly. When people have repeated panic attacks that they can't predict (they come out of the blue) and can't control, this can lead to panic disorder. If you have had two or more episodes of panic within a short period of time (1 to 2 months), and live in fear of further panic attacks, you should see a mental health professional. A common consequence of having unexpected panics is to develop a pattern of avoidance; usually people avoid any situation in which they do not feel safe. This is called agoraphobia and is also a reason to seek professional treatment.

Panic attacks are also associated with phobias, which refer to fears of specific things. The most disabling phobia is social phobia, in which the person lives in dread of being evaluated negatively by others. Other phobias include intense fears and avoidance of animals, blood, heights, water, flying, and a host of other things. As with depression, there are a number of medical and psychological treatments that can be very effective for treating panic disorders.

Generalized anxiety refers to the tendency to worry to excess about most everything (big and small) most of the time. These people are sometimes called worrywarts. All of us worry, but there is usually a realistic threat causing the worry. People who have generalized anxiety disorder spend most of their time worrying about things that are minor as well as major and are generally unable to control or dismiss their worries. Subjective distress and interference with normal activities are the keys to deciding whether your worries are excessive. Often professional advice is needed to accurately diagnose generalized anxiety.

Two other anxiety disorders should be mentioned for the sake of completeness. However, they are relatively uncommon and are not often associated with irritable bowel. Obsessive-compulsive disorder involves either anxiety-provoking thoughts that can't be controlled (called obsessions or ruminations) or behaviors that make no sense and are compulsively repeated (such as excessive hand washing, checking locks, counting objects, etc.). Post-traumatic stress disorder can develop after the experience of a trauma, such as being raped, robbed, assaulted, or being in a bad car accident. The symptoms include reliving the trauma in one's mind, general anxiety, intrusive thoughts, and feelings of detachment from life in general. If you think you may have either of these problems, talk to your family doctor about a more detailed assessment.

Substance Abuse Disorders

Finally, we would like to mention the problem of substance abuse. In an attempt to cope with life problems, such as irritable bowel, some people turn to drugs or medication.

The damaging effects of drinking problems are well known. What's less recognized is the different effect alcohol has on women versus men. In general, alcohol affects women more because of their size and body composition. Many women don't label themselves as having an alcohol problem when drinking 3 or 4 drinks per day, but this can be equivalent to 6 to 8 drinks in a man.

Many people who are dead-set against street drugs can develop problems with prescription medication. This is especially true for managing pain. Many of the powerful painkillers are very addictive (such as Demerol).

There are a wide variety of effective means to tackle substance abuse problems. Before that, though, you need to recognize if you or a loved one has a substance abuse problem. Many physicians use the following CAGE questionnaire to assess the presence of a drinking problem. You might also ask someone you trust (who doesn't have a problem themselves) if they are concerned about your substance use.

Is Alcohol a Problem?

Check the statements that are true for you. If you check 2 or more, it is likely that you have a drinking problem and you should seek help.

_____ **C** Have you felt the need to Cut down on your drinking?

_____ **A** Have you felt Annoyed when people comment on your drinking?

_____ **G** Have you felt Guilty about your drinking?

_____ **E** Have you had a drink in the morning to get rid of a hangover or steady your nerves (an Eye-opener)?

Chapter Eleven

Working With
Your Doctor

When irritable bowel symptoms first surface, a doctor will focus on the question: Is something dangerous causing these symptoms? Once irritable bowel is diagnosed, the focus turns to managing those symptoms and responding to problems.

In many ways, having an irritable bowel forces you to become your own doctor. It is up to you to control your symptoms by what you eat, when you eat, and how you act and react to life's daily stresses. Your physician will be the person you turn to for expert advice and to decide if symptom changes warrant further tests.

Few doctors receive much training in managing irritable bowel, especially concerning nutrition strategies (that's why this book is so important). Even so, you should contact your doctor if your symptoms change or if you experience problems not associated with an irritable bowel, such as blood in the stool (see chapters 1 and 2).

To get the most from your doctor's appointments, there are a few things to remember:

If you have a specific concern, tell your doctor immediately. Some patients don't mention what's really on their mind until they are putting on their coat and heading to the door. By waiting until the last moment, your doctor may not recognize it as a major concern or will assume you just want a quick reassurance.

If you are afraid you have cancer, say so. Speaking the word "cancer" does not mean you will get it. We mention cancer specifically because it is very common for people with irritable bowel to have this fear. Doctors know the symptoms of cancer and can quickly evaluate your symptoms and provide reassurance if they do not indicate cancer. If, however, you do not express your fear about cancer (or any other symptom), your doctor will assume that you know the symptoms are not dangerous. Internalizing concerns often causes distress, which can contribute to the worsening of your symptoms. Many patients see improvement simply by being reassured that they do not have cancer or colitis or other dangerous bowel diseases.

Resist being intimidated by your doctor. Doctors are often very busy and may give you the impression that they are having to rush to see you. To help avoid being flustered, try to jot down your questions so that you are sure you won't forget them. It will also help to bring your symptom list from chapter 2.

Remember, there are no stupid questions. Your doctor has heard them all and can most likely address any concern, but you need to voice them. Being yourself and speaking frankly about your concerns goes a long way in building a trusting relationship with your doctor. This is crucial. If you do not believe what your doctor tells you, then you will not be reassured, and you will probably end up seeing other doctors unnecessarily.

Seek out a doctor who listens to and answers your questions, then continue seeing that doctor. Doctors know when they don't have the right skills to manage a problem and will refer you to other specialists if necessary. Seeing many doctors for second opinions usually results in unnecessary tests, and little is done to help you better manage your symptoms.

Make sure you understand your doctor's instructions. If your doctor gives you advice, or asks you to do something, it is important to clarify what she wants you to do. You should understand why you are taking a medication, what it is supposed to do, and any side effects to watch for. Only by making sure you understand your doctor's instructions will it be possible for you to work effectively with your doctor.

A Patient/Doctor Dialogue

Much of your discussion with your doctor will probably be related to the symptoms of irritable bowel. We thought it would be helpful to review what we know about those symptoms by presenting a dialogue that covers common questions and comments from patients.

> Patient: When my bowels work, the stool often starts off as solid or even hard, then it becomes increasingly loose after I have gone to the bathroom several times over an hour or two. I have severe cramps in the lower belly and often feel tired and drained. Also, I sometimes feel hot and break out in a sweat.

> Doctor: An irritable bowel will frequently cause this pattern of defecation. In fact, it can be used as a diagnostic tool. What you have described are three of the six typical irritable bowel symptoms. You start with solid stool that becomes increasingly loose and more frequent and is associated with the abdominal cramping pain. After your bowel motion you also notice that you have a feeling of incomplete rectal emptying. And if you look at the bowel motion you may see a slimy substance in the stool. This substance, which we call mucus, is a normal lubricant produced by the bowel. There may be times that instead of stool you just pass this slimy substance with little or no stool.

> You will feel tired and drained with sweating because your body has reacted to the diarrhea by activating the "sympathetic nervous system." These are the nerves that prime the heart to pump the blood to the body faster, which often causes a flushing sensation that makes you feel warm. Sweating occurs to regulate the body's temperature so that it does not increase with the increased blood flow to the body tissues. These are normal sensations called the flight-or-fight response that our body does when it feels threatened. It is a normal response and can occur with diarrhea or other unpleasant symptoms. It is not in your head. These are normal body sensations even though they can feel unpleasant and alarming.

> Patient: I usually feel so bloated after eating that on most days I eat just one big meal. I skip breakfast and rarely have lunch because I know eating makes the

bloating worse. I am often constipated and unable to have a bowel motion more than twice a week.

Doctor: Healthy eating habits and trying to keep a routine eating schedule will be important for your bowel. First, you are not eating in a way that will help to improve your constipation. Breakfast is probably the most important meal of the day because your large bowel is most active in the morning when you wake up. Eating breakfast will further stimulate your bowel and greatly increase your chances of having more regular bowel motions.

Abdominal bloating tends to be worse if you eat just one meal a day, especially if it's a large meal, which is usually the case. Bloating also tends to be worse later in the day. To help ease your bloating, try to eat smaller meals more frequently and earlier in the day. Make breakfast your larger meal of the day and supper a light snack. (See chapter 5 for a more comprehensive guide on how to manage gas and bloating symptoms.)

Patient: Doctor, I've noticed undigested food when I have gone to the bathroom, especially when I have diarrhea. I am not too surprised about seeing corn, but sometimes I see tomato skins, seeds, or other pieces of fruits and vegetables.

Doctor: What you are describing is normal. Fibrous foods such as vegetables and fruits are not completely digested even though their nutrients are extracted by the intestines. Undigested food is just easier to spot in diarrheal stool. Corn can be seen even in normal solid stool because of its bright yellow color, but other undigested foods are in the stool as well. It is *not* normal to see meat fibers and fat in the stool. This indicates a problem with food digestion.

At times you may notice that the normal mucus present in stool looks like fat globules. This can be confusing, but it is rare for the body to be having trouble absorbing fat and not lose weight. If you are losing weight, further testing can be done on the stool to confirm a problem with fat malabsorption.

Patient: I am worried that I may have a digestion problem. My stool often floats. Doesn't that mean fat isn't being digested properly?

Doctor: Sometimes when there is fat malabsorption the stool floats, but most of the time a floating stool means gas in the intestine has been trapped in the solid stool, allowing it to float. Stools that float are normal and nothing to worry about.

Patient: Sometimes when I have diarrhea, after several bowel motions, my stool turns green. Is this serious?

Doctor: Stool gets its normal brown color when bacteria change unabsorbed bile in the intestine to a yellow/brown pigment. If you have diarrhea, the stool can pass through the gut too quickly for this color change to occur. The only abnormal colors for stool are red, black, and an off-white or clay-colored stool. Very light colored stools can be due to bile not getting into the intestines in the first place. This is usually accompanied by jaundice (a yellow color to the skin and the whites of the eyes) and urine that is dark yellow or almost brown (tea-colored). Stool that is red or black can be due to internal bleeding and blood loss. The source of a red color is obvious; the black color occurs because bacteria in the gut change the red color in blood to a black pigment. Tests can be done on the stool if it is black to confirm there is blood present.

Further tests should always be done if the stool is red or black to find the cause of bleeding. This is not normal and is not part of an irritable bowel. Some causes of bleeding can be minor, such as hemorrhoids or an anal fissure (a split of the skin lining the anal opening to the rectum). You should always tell your doctor if you see bleeding so that the true cause can be found.

Some medications can also turn the bowel motions black. The most common is iron medication, but if you are taking iron for anemia or "low blood," tests should first be done to check the stool for blood (even if the stool has a normal brown color) to be sure the anemia is not due to blood loss from the gut. Licorice and medications with bismuth such as Pepto-Bismol can also cause a black discoloration of the stool.

Patient: I have been looking up information on I.B.S. on the Internet. One medication was advertised that will regulate my bowels and was touted as having all "natural ingredients." I have also read claims that I.B.S. is not a real disease but a mental disorder.

Doctor: When seeking out further information, particularly on the Internet, you should be very careful about the claims of products for treating medical conditions. Many products with "all natural ingredients" that claim to "help" the bowels contain laxatives that are classed as stimulants. These come from plant

extracts; the most common ones are Senna and Cas-
cara sagrada, which can actually damage the bowel
and aggravate constipation if taken daily for long
periods of time. The manufacturer can correctly claim
the product is all natural, since the extract from the
plants has laxative properties in the bowel. Other
plants, such as deadly nightshade, are known to be
deadly poisons, yet they could also carry the same
healthy-sounding label, "all natural." If you plan to
buy such products, it is as always, Buyer Beware! If
you are not sure, bring in the ingredient list, and we
can check it over to see if there are any potentially
harmful substances in the product.

As for the information on the Internet, remember
that anyone can say anything they want, even if it is
incorrect. As we have outlined already, it was thought
that irritable bowel was a psychological disorder. We
now know this to be incorrect. Psychological factors
such as stress and anxiety will worsen your irritable
bowel symptoms, but they are not the cause of your
symptoms.

Afterword

We truly hope that you have found *I.B.S. Relief* useful. But before you return the book to its place on the shelf, we have two suggestions:

First, sit down and write yourself a letter. That's right, write a letter to yourself! Let us explain. We want you to write a letter to the person you were before starting this book. Knowing what you do now, advise yourself on how to handle irritable bowel. Identify the symptoms you began with, and how they were distressing to you. Go on to list what you have learned about those symptoms and your body. Identify your dietary and psychological triggers and then tell yourself what interventions you found helpful (and how you implemented them). Then put this letter inside the front cover.

If sometime in the future (6 months? 6 years?) you begin to re-experience irritable bowel, reread the letter. We have found that if you capture in your own words your experience in treating irritable bowel, it will be tremendously helpful if you should need to treat yourself again in the future. Combined with this book, you should be in good shape to prevent future problems.

The second thing we suggest is that you complete another symptom diary, as you did in chapter 2 (see page 19). On the following pages, extra diary forms are presented. Once you have completed the diary again, compare it to your first one. Not only will this show you how far you have come, it will also point out remaining issues that may need special attention in the future.

One final point: We thought you might find it useful if we listed what we feel are the top 10 things to do to manage irritable bowel. We hope you find the list on page 143 helpful.

Thanks for taking the time to work through *I.B.S. Relief.* It is our hope that we have empowered you to reduce the control that irritable bowel symptoms can have on your life.

> Dawn Burstall
> Michael Vallis
> Geoffrey Turnbull

ENLARGE THIS RECORD TO 200% ON YOUR COPIER

Symptom Diary

	Monday	Tuesday	Wednesday
Date and Time			
Symptoms and Severity (1=not at all severe; 10=extremely severe)			
Food Triggers			
Stress Level (1=no stress; 10=extreme stress)			
Feelings and Worries			

ENLARGE THIS RECORD TO 200% ON YOUR COPIER

Symptom Diary

	Thursday	Friday	Saturday	Sunday
Date and Time				
Symptoms and Severity (1=not at all severe; 10=extremely severe)				
Food Triggers				
Stress Level (1=no stress; 10=extreme stress)				
Feelings and Worries				

The Top 10 Tips for Living With an Irritable Bowel

1. Remember that your bowel is normal—just "irritable."

2. Your bowel will thrive on routine (eat meals regularly and get adequate sleep).

3. Identify and limit foods that trigger symptoms.

4. Eat plenty of fiber (20 to 35 grams) and drink 8 glasses of caffeine-free liquid each day.

5. Adjust your diet to your symptoms.

6. Identify sources of stress.

7. Practice relaxation strategies.

8. Set your priorities realistically.

9. Accept, adapt, and learn to let go.

10. Work with your doctor; express concerns.

How Does the Gut Work?
A Quick Guide

The intestinal tract is an often overlooked and underappreci-ated part of the body. Clearly the brain, heart, and a few other body organs rate higher on the list of "importance." How-ever, the gut is vital for the nutritional support of the body and, as we will outline, is very important in maintaining health.

The word *gut* refers to the intestines (bowels) and can include the stomach, esophagus, and the other digestive organs, the pan-creas, and the bile system. The gut serves several purposes. It is designed to take in nourishment and process it to be absorbed and used by the body. Because the gut takes in food and nourish-ment from the surrounding environment, it is designed to pro-vide an infection barrier between the environment and the internal workings of the body. The gut is also important for obtaining fluid and regulating the excretion of fluid and nutrients so that the body can maximize its fluid and calorie sources.

The gut is organized into three areas: esophagus, stomach, and intestines. The esophagus is essentially a food pipe that transmits food from the mouth to the stomach. The stomach then serves to liquefy and break down food products into a more digestible liq-uid mush. Digestion actually begins in the mouth when enzymes in saliva mix with food to help break down starch carbohydrates. While saliva helps to lubricate food, teeth are used to break the food into smaller chunks, which facilitates further food break-down and digestion in the stomach.

The stomach does not truly digest food but secretes acid to help break down some of the components of food so that they will be more easily digested in the small intestine. Perhaps most importantly, though, the stomach serves as a reservoir for food, allowing large quantities of food to be eaten intermittently. Though stomach acid helps break down food particles, it is not required to digest food. We know this because individuals do live without a stomach while maintaining their nutritional status. Others live with a stomach that is unable to produce acid and also have no problems digesting food. (These individuals, however, are much more likely to acquire intestinal infection.) One of the most important properties of stomach acid is to kill harmful organisms, particularly bacteria and parasites as well as viruses. In addition, acid in the stomach helps the absorption of iron from vegetables and grains (not meats). The acid-producing cells in the stomach also produce a factor needed for vitamin B_{12} absorption in the intestine.

Once the stomach has churned food into a liquid pulp or mush, small quantities are gradually released through a special muscle valve opening between the stomach and small intestine called the pylorus (figure 1). This releases small quantities of food into the small intestine, where alkali or bicarbonate is secreted to neutralize stomach acid. This is facilitated by bicarbonate secretions from the pancreas and bile duct, which also empty into the first part of the small intestine, called the duodenum. Secretions from the pancreas also contain enzymes needed to digest food into its component parts.

Bile from the liver is extremely important in the digestion of food, particularly the digestion of fat, which is the most difficult foodstuff for the intestine to break down and absorb. A number of hormones are released in the duodenum, which help to stimulate secretions from the pancreas and bile from the gallbladder and the liver. These same hormones—along with the electrical and muscle control of the gut—change as soon as food starts to enter the small intestine. This prepares the small intestine for its specific muscle contraction pattern or rhythm that mixes food and intestinal juice, further facilitating the breakdown of food and maximizing absorption (figure 2).

Figure 1

The Upper
Gastrointestinal Tract

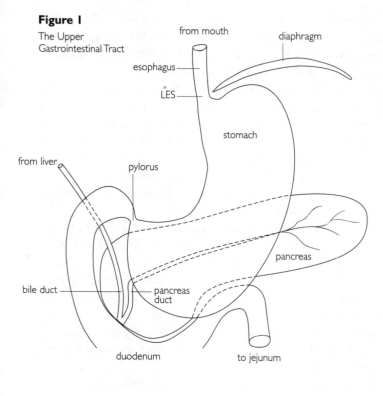

Figure 2

The Small Intestine

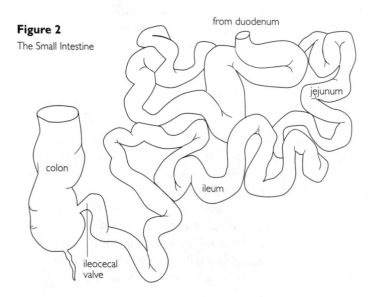

Large quantities of fluid and salts, or "electrolytes," mix with food to keep it in a liquid state. As food moves through the small intestine, it is gradually broken down by the pancreatic enzymes and the enzymes lining the small intestine. In the presence of bile salts (which break the fat globules into smaller, more soluble globules called micelles), the enzymes from the pancreas can then digest the fat so that it can be absorbed into the body. The food that is absorbed from the intestine enters the bloodstream and is transported to the liver, which cleanses the blood and recirculates the nutrients into the bloodstream. The nutrients then flow to the rest of the body, providing what the body's cells need for their metabolism and function.

The small intestine is clearly a vital organ for life. Its huge surface area, estimated at the size of a football field, allows close contact between the food and the cells lining the small intestine, which absorb the component parts of the food. Essentially, food can be broken down into four components: (1) carbohydrates are broken down into sugars; (2) proteins are broken down into amino acids; (3) fat is broken down into fatty acids and glycerol; and, (4) specific vitamins and minerals that are necessary for health are extracted from foods.

Under normal circumstances, all of the carbohydrate sources such as starch and sugars are absorbed along with all of the protein and 95 percent of the fat ingested. This leaves one large group of foodstuffs that have not been mentioned but are very important components of the diet: fiber.

Fiber's Role

Fiber is present in whole grains, fruits, vegetables, nuts, seeds, and dried beans (not meats or dairy products). Fiber is usually made up of complex carbohydrates or sugar residues that are **not** digestible by the enzymes in the small intestine and pancreas. However, fiber can be broken down by bacterial enzymes, and this is the next step in the digestion process.

Fiber is usually not released from the stomach until after a meal is completed and all digestible substances have been absorbed. The gut then changes its pattern of muscle contraction so that residues containing the fiber are emptied from the stomach and passed through the small intestine relatively quickly and into the large intestine undigested. The gut functions this way, since the fiber may interfere with the normal absorption of food-stuffs. Still, fiber is absolutely crucial to normal large-gut function. In the presence of bacteria that normally live in the large bowel, fiber is digested by the bacterial enzymes, and nutrients from the breakdown are absolutely crucial for the normal health of the lining cells of the large bowel. Gas can also be a by-product of this bacterial digestion of fiber. A diet lacking in fiber will often lead to further problems in large-bowel activity.

The large intestine (figure 3) primarily absorbs the liquid presented to it by the small intestine after the digestible substances have been absorbed in the small intestine. The colon, or large intestine, reabsorbs the liquid from the small intestine to form solid stool waste. Much of the stool is, in fact, made up of bacterial waste because the colon normally contains large quantities of bacteria. Once the content of the stool has been made into a more solid product, it is then transported into the lower large intestine, or rectum, and emptying of the stool occurs when you feel the stool in the rectum.

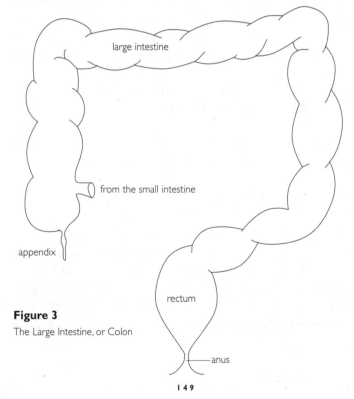

large intestine

from the small intestine

appendix

rectum

Figure 3

The Large Intestine, or Colon

anus

Gut Timing

A common point of confusion is how long it normally takes foods to move through the gut. Food passes through the esophagus in a matter of seconds and is usually emptied to the stomach in under a minute. It may take as long as three or four hours after a meal before the stomach empties. It may take even longer, though, depending on the size and content of the meal. Generally, high-fat meals take much longer for the stomach to empty. While the stomach is slowly emptying the food into the small intestine, the small intestine will take four to six hours to finish digesting a meal.

When you consider the time it takes to digest meals, for most people who eat three meals a day, the body reaches its fasting state (when there is no food left in the intestines to digest) mostly at night. This is important to note because it is only after the small intestine has emptied that fiber residues are emptied into the large intestine. It can take two to three days before material is finally packaged into stool and emptied from the rectum.

So why do people usually experience an urge to pass stool an hour or two after eating, or daily, or every two days? This is because normal nerve connections and reflexes trigger the large intestine to increase its activity, particularly first thing in the morning so that the remaining food residues (stool) that have been stored for a day or two are moved into the rectum and evacuated. Colonic function is most active first thing in the morning, after waking. This means that to achieve a regular bowel habit, it is best to eat some food in the morning to help maximize this stimulation of the colon, which results in more regular defecation.

A "Thoughtful" Gut

The digestion process is incredibly complex and, although simplified here, is still not as well understood as it should be. Nevertheless, the gut appears to be able to work quite well on its own due to a "little brain." Complex nerve connections direct the gut through specific muscle contraction sequences depending on whether or not there is food in the intestine. Some evidence regarding irritable bowel shows that the functions of this "little brain" may be disturbed in its coordination, which, not surprisingly, can lead to symptoms typical of an irritable bowel.

Canada's Food Guide

C anada's Food Guide to Healthy Eating (see pages 154–55) is represented very differently than the American Food Guide Pyramid (see page 28); however, the content—and advice— is very similar. In fact, Canadians using this book and learning about the Food Pyramid are following National Canadian standards as well.

Canada's "rainbow" design features four food groups with fruits and vegetables combined into one food group. The American Food Guide Pyramid, on the other hand, puts fruits and vegetables in separate groups. Another slight difference is that Fats, Oils, and Sweets on the Pyramid tip are called "Other Foods" in Canada's Food Guide.

The number of servings recommended for each food group differ in some food groups; the major difference being the recommended servings from the dairy groups. The American Food Guide Pyramid recommends 3 servings of milk products per day until the age of 24 and for pregnant and breast-feeding women. Canada's Food Guide recommends 3 to 4 servings of milk products until the age of 17 and for pregnant and breast-feeding women. Serving sizes differ slightly on a few items between the food guides but not significantly.

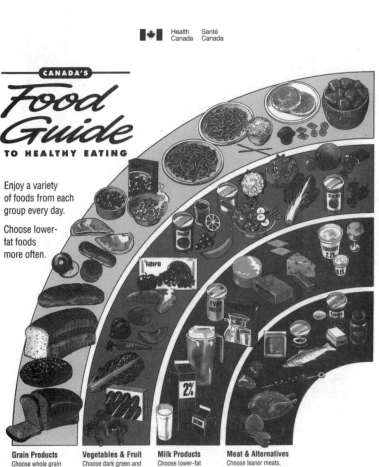

Health Santé
Canada Canada

CANADA'S
Food Guide
TO HEALTHY EATING

Enjoy a variety
of foods from each
group every day.

Choose lower-
fat foods
more often.

Grain Products
Choose whole grain
and enriched
products more
often.

Vegetables & Fruit
Choose dark green and
orange vegetables and
orange fruit more often.

Milk Products
Choose lower-fat
milk products more
often.

Meat & Alternatives
Choose leaner meats,
poultry and fish, as well
as dried peas, beans and
lentils more often.

Canadä

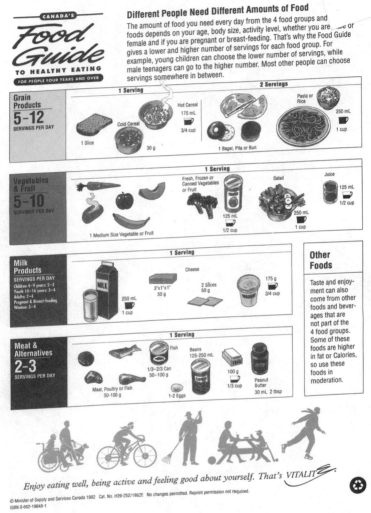

CANADA'S Food Guide
TO HEALTHY EATING
FOR PEOPLE FOUR YEARS AND OVER

Different People Need Different Amounts of Food

The amount of food you need every day from the 4 food groups and foods depends on your age, body size, activity level, whether you are male or female and if you are pregnant or breast-feeding. That's why the Food Guide gives a lower and higher number of servings for each food group. For example, young children can choose the lower number of servings, while male teenagers can go to the higher number. Most other people can choose servings somewhere in between.

Grain Products
5-12
SERVINGS PER DAY

1 Serving — Cold Cereal 30 g, 1 Slice, Hot Cereal 175 mL 3/4 cup
2 Servings — 1 Bagel, Pita or Bun, Pasta or Rice 250 mL 1 cup

Vegetables & Fruit
5-10
SERVINGS PER DAY

1 Serving — 1 Medium Size Vegetable or Fruit, Fresh, Frozen or Canned Vegetables or Fruit 125 mL 1/2 cup, Salad 250 mL 1 cup, Juice 125 mL 1/2 cup

Milk Products
SERVINGS PER DAY
Children 4–9 years: 2–3
Youth 10–16 years: 3–4
Adults: 2–4
Pregnant & Breast-feeding Women: 3–4

1 Serving — MILK 250 mL 1 cup, Cheese 3"x1"x1" 50 g, 2 Slices 50 g, Yogurt 175 g 3/4 cup

Meat & Alternatives
2-3
SERVINGS PER DAY

1 Serving — Meat, Poultry or Fish 50–100 g, Fish 1/3–2/3 Can 50–100 g, 1-2 Eggs, Beans 125–250 mL, Tofu 100 g 1/3 cup, Peanut Butter 30 mL 2 tbsp

Other Foods

Taste and enjoyment can also come from other foods and beverages that are not part of the 4 food groups. Some of these foods are higher in fat or Calories, so use these foods in moderation.

Enjoy eating well, being active and feeling good about yourself. That's VITALITY

© Minister of Supply and Services Canada 1992 Cat. No. H39-252/1992E No changes permitted. Reprint permission not required.
ISBN 0-662-19648-1

High-Fiber, Low-Fat Recipes

Before presenting a few high-fiber, low-fat recipes, here are some pointers on how to increase the fiber and reduce the fat content in existing recipes.

To increase the fiber (insoluble) content:

- Use half whole-wheat and half white flour in baked items.
- Add natural bran to pancakes, muffins, cakes, hot cereal, stews, casseroles, soups, and meatloaf.

To decrease the fat content:

- Decrease the fat in your recipes by a third to a half. For example, a muffin recipe that calls for 1/2 cup (120 ml) of margarine can be cut back to 1/4 cup (60 ml) with little, if any, change to the finished product.
- Add moisture to recipes by adding fruit like applesauce or canned pumpkin. Applesauce does not add flavor, whereas pumpkin contributes a unique flavor. By adding applesauce and pumpkin, you can cut back on the sugar in the recipe as well. Adding fruit may extend the cooking time by 2 to 3 minutes.
- Reduce the fat, saturated fat, and cholesterol in your recipes by decreasing the egg yolk content by half. For example, if a recipe calls for 2 whole eggs, use 1 whole egg and 1 egg white.

The following recipes were developed mostly from existing recipes using the foregoing simple guidelines. While the recipes are reduced in fat and have added fiber, some do not meet the strict definition of "low-fat" (3 grams or less of fat per serving) or "high fiber" (5 grams or more of fiber per serving).

Grainy Gingerbread Cake

1/2 cup packed brown sugar	3/4 cup all-purpose flour
1/4 cup margarine	1/2 cup natural (baker's) bran
1 egg	1 tsp. baking soda
1 egg white	1 tsp. baking powder
1 cup unsweetened applesauce	2 tsp. ground ginger
1/2 cup molasses	1 tsp. ground cinnamon
3/4 cup whole-wheat flour	1/2 tsp. salt

1. In a bowl, using an electric mixer, beat brown sugar and margarine until smooth.

2. Add egg and egg white, beating well after each addition. Add applesauce and molasses, beat until smooth.

3. Combine flour, natural bran, baking soda, baking powder, ginger, cinnamon, and salt; gradually beat into sugar and egg mixture, beating for 2 to 3 minutes.

4. Transfer to 8-inch (20 cm) lightly greased and floured square cake pan. Bake at 350° F (180° C) for 40 minutes.

5. Pour fruit-flavored low-fat yogurt over gingerbread before serving (optional).

Makes 12 servings

Per Serving (cake only): Calories 170, Carbohydrates 31 g, Fiber 2.3 g, Fat 4 g, Saturated fat 1 g, Cholesterol 18 mg, Protein 2 g, Sodium 231 mg

Irish Soda Bread

2 cups whole-wheat flour	1 tsp. salt
1 cup white flour	2 Tbsp. sesame seeds (optional)
1 cup natural bran	3 Tbsp. poppy seeds (optional)
1 cup quick oats	1/4 cup liquid honey
1 1/2 tsp. baking soda	2 cups buttermilk or low-fat plain
1 tsp. baking powder	yogurt

1. Mix dry ingredients.

2. Combine honey with dry ingredients. Make a well in the center of dry mixture.

3. Add buttermilk or yogurt and mix until fully combined.

4. Place in pie plate. Make a cross on the top with the sharp edge of a knife.

5. Bake at 375° F (190° C) for 40 to 50 minutes.

Makes 16 servings

Per Serving: Calories 155, Carbohydrates 35 g, Fiber 4.2 g, Fat 3 g, Saturated fat 0.5 g, Cholesterol 1 mg, Protein 5.8 g, Sodium 238 mg

Apple Crisp

1/4 cup white sugar	1/4 cup white flour
2 Tbsp. white flour	1/4 cup brown sugar
1 tsp. grated lemon rind	1 tsp. cinnamon
6 cups peeled and sliced apples	1/4 cup soft margarine
3/4 cup quick rolled oats	1/2 cup very high fiber wheat
1/4 cup whole-wheat flour	bran cereal

1. Combine sugar, flour, and lemon rind, mix well.

2. Add apple and mix, pour into 8-cup (2 liter) baking dish.

3. Combine rolled oats, whole wheat and white flour, brown sugar, cinnamon. Blend in margarine with a pastry cutter. Mix in very high fiber bran cereal.

4. Sprinkle over apple mixture.

5. Bake at 375° F (190° C) for 35 to 40 minutes.

Makes 8 servings

Per Serving: Calories 250, Carbohydrates 49 g, Fiber 3.1 g, Fat 6.8 g, Saturated fat 1 g, Cholesterol 0, Protein 2.7 g, Sodium 36 mg

Whole-Wheat Pizza Crust

2 cups warm water	1/4 cup vegetable oil
2 tsp. sugar	2 1/2 cups whole-wheat flour
2 envelopes fast-rise yeast	2 cups white flour

1. Dissolve sugar in warm water in a large bowl. Sprinkle yeast into water and let stand 10 minutes.

2. Stir oil into yeast mixture. Stir in whole-wheat flour. Then add more whole-wheat and white flour, mixing until dough can be gathered in a slightly sticky ball.

3. On a lightly floured surface, knead dough for about 5 minutes or until smooth and elastic.

4. Cut dough in half, cover with wax paper, and let rest for 30 to 40 minutes.

5. On a floured surface, roll out each piece of dough to about 12 inches (30 cm) in diameter.

6. Transfer to lightly greased pizza rounds and carefully pull and stretch with fingers to make fit pan. Let rest for about 20 to 30 minutes more before adding toppings. For a thicker crust, let rest for 30 to 40 minutes.

7. Spread with tomato sauce, your favorite vegetables, and low-fat cheese just before baking.

8. Bake at 450° F (225° C) for 15 to 20 minutes.

Makes two 12-inch (30 cm) pizza rounds.
Total of 16 servings, each serving = 1/8 of one pizza.

Per Serving (crust only): Calories 159, Carbohydrates 36 g, Fiber 2.8 g, Fat 4 g, Saturated fat 0.6 g, Cholesterol 0, Protein 4.2 g, Sodium 1 mg

Blueberry Whole-Wheat Pancakes

1 cup white flour	1 1/2 cups 1% milk
1 cup whole-wheat flour	2 Tbsp. vegetable oil
1/4 tsp. cinnamon	1 egg
1/2 tsp. salt	1 cup blueberries

1. Mix dry ingredients.

2. Beat liquids together and add to dry ingredients, blend until there are no lumps.

3. Keep in refrigerator for a couple of hours or overnight.

4. When ready to prepare, stir in blueberries.

5. Brush skillet or griddle with oil or use nonstick pan, set burner to medium.

6. Pour batter using 1/4 cup for each pancake.

7. When underside is brown and bubbles break on top (after 1 to 2 minutes), turn pancake over and cook for 30 to 60 seconds or until second side is golden brown.

Makes 12 servings

Per Serving: Calories 118, Carbohydrates 27 g, Fiber 1.8 g, Fat 3.4 g, Saturated fat 0.7 g, Cholesterol 18.5 mg, Protein 3.5 g, Sodium 117 mg

Branana Muffins

1 egg	1/4 cup vegetable oil
1 cup ripe bananas, mashed	2 Tbsp. molasses
1 cup very high fiber wheat	1 cup white flour
bran cereal	1 cup whole wheat flour
3/4 cup 1% milk	1 tsp. baking powder
1/2 cup brown sugar	1/2 tsp. salt

1. Beat egg in bowl with fork. Blend in banana, cereal, milk, sugar, oil, and molasses.

2. Combine dry ingredients in a large bowl. Make a well in the center.

3. Stir liquid ingredients into dry ingredients, stirring just until moistened.

4. Spoon into lightly greased muffin cups, generously fill to the top.

5. Bake at 400° F (200° C) for 18 to 20 minutes or until golden brown.

Makes 12 large muffins

Per Serving: Calories 197, Carbohydrates 40 g, Fiber 3.5 g, Fat 6 g, Saturated fat 1 g, Cholesterol 18 mg, Protein 5.6 g, Sodium 267 mg

Peanut Butter Bran Muffins

3/4 cup all-purpose flour

3/4 cup whole-wheat flour

1 Tbsp. baking powder

1/2 tsp. salt

1 cup very high fiber wheat
bran creal

1 cup 1% milk

1 egg

1/2 cup peanut butter

1/4 cup milk

1/4 cup honey

1. Combine flour, sugar, baking powder, and salt in a large mixing bowl. Mix well and make a well in the center.

2. Combine cereal with 1 cup of milk in medium bowl.

3. Combine egg and peanut butter, and add 1/4 cup milk, and honey.

4. Combine peanut butter mixture with cereal and milk mixture. Pour into well of dry ingredients. Stir only enough to moisten.

5. Fill lightly greased muffin tins 3/4 full.

6. Bake at 400° F (200° C) for 17 to 18 minutes.

Makes 12 muffins

Per Serving: Calories 167, Carbohydrates 25 g, Fiber 2.8 g, Fat 6.2 g, Saturated fat 0.6 g, Cholesterol 19 mg, Protein 6.4 g, Sodium 317 mg

Pumpkin Bran Muffins

1/4 cup vegetable oil
1/2 cup brown sugar
1/4 cup molasses
1 egg
1 egg white
3/4 cup 1% milk
1 cup canned pumpkin

1 1/4 cups white flour
1 1/2 tsp. baking powder
1/2 tsp. baking soda
3/4 tsp. salt
1 1/2 cups natural wheat bran
1/2 cup raisins

1. Mix vegetable oil, brown sugar, and molasses.

2. Add egg and egg white, beat after each addition.

3. Stir in milk and canned pumpkin.

4. Combine dry ingredients and raisins.

5. Combine liquid and dry ingredients, mixing as little as possible.

6. Fill lightly greased muffin cups 3/4 full.

7. Bake at 400° F (200° C) for 17 to 20 minutes.

Makes 12 muffins

Per Serving: Calories 193, Carbohydrates 45.6 g, Fiber 4.4 g, Fat 5.7 g, Saturated fat 0.1 g, Cholesterol 18 mg, Protein 3.4 g, Sodium 245 mg

Metric Conversion Chart

1/4 cup = 60 ml

1/3 cup = 75 ml

1/2 cup = 120 ml

2/3 cup = 150 ml

3/4 cup = 175 ml

1 cup = 250 ml

1 1/4 cups = 300 ml

1 1/2 cups = 375 ml

1/2 tsp. = 2 ml

1 tsp. = 5 ml

2 tsp. = 10 ml

1 Tbsp. = 15 ml

Additional Resources

The following books and organizations may help to supplement some of the information we have presented in this book as well as provide more details about how the gut functions.

1. Thompson, W. Grant. *Gut Reactions: Understanding Symptoms of the Digestive Tract.* Plenum Press, New York & London, 1989.

2. Janowitz, Henry D. *Your Gut Feelings.* Oxford University Press, New York & Oxford, 1994.

3. Guillory, Gerard. *IBS: A Doctor's Plan for Chronic Digestive Troubles.* Hartley & Marks, Point Roberts, Washington, 1996.

4. *The American Dietetic Association's Complete Food & Nutrition Guide.* Chronimed Publishing, Minneapolis, 1996.

5. *Consumer Reports* magazine, which often prints food nutrition information.

6. International Foundation for Functional Gastrointestinal Disorders (IFFGD). P.O. Box 17864, Milwaukee, WI 53217. Tel: (414) 964-1799.

7. The National Digestive Diseases Information Clearinghouse. 2 Information Way, Bethesda, MD 20892-3570. Tel: (301) 654-3810.

Index

Charts are in italics.